Positive Options
Complex Regional Pain Sy

"Ms. Juris has written a wonderful, readable, hope-filled book for individuals and families struggling with a too often intractable foe."

— Jim Broatch, MSW, executive director
Reflex Sympathetic Dystrophy Syndrome Association of America

"Finally, what those living with CRPS have needed for so long—an inspirational, positive voice that speaks to us calmly, confidentially, wisely, and equally comforting."

— Helen Small, president
PARC, Promoting Awareness of RSD and CRPS in Canada

"This book is an unabridged trek to Planet CRPS and beyond. Inside this book, you will find the most eclectic collection of sometimes wild, sometimes customary coping techniques that spawn a complete reinvention of the self. More than simply a 'self-help' manual, the book is a testament to the enduring nature of the human spirit. It provides lifesaving wisdom and is not afraid to examine the brutal difficulties of constant pain and lost independence. It far outreaches expectation in providing pragmatic information and fostering real-life hope."

— Sosha Devi, Yoga for Chronic Pain Project and
(formerly) The American Pain Foundation, Baltimore, Maryland

"As a recovered CRPS patient myself and a psychologist who specializes in CRPS and pain management, I am delighted to say that this highly practical and action-oriented book is the most comprehensive storehouse of pain relief I've seen around.... Bravo, Elena Juris, for inspiring us all!"

— Phyliss Shanken, MA, psychologist, director of psychological services
INTROSPECT of BuxMont, Colmar, Pennsylvania

"I can think of no diseases other than reflex sympathetic dystrophy where patient participation in the management is more important.... Elena Juris's book is not only an inspiration to those who suffer from this disease, it also inspires caregivers and health-care professionals who participate in their treatment."

— Harry F. L. Pollett, MD, FRCPC
medical director, Non-Malignant Pain Clinic
Northside General Hospital, North Sydney, Nova Scotia

"Elena does a wonderful job demonstrating how, in addition to skilled physical therapy, multiple complementary therapies play a critical role in the individualized rehabilitation of RSD/CRPS."

— Stephanie Gilliam, MPT
Arlington, Virginia

"The author validates the emotional struggles of those with RSD, as well as their medical and practical needs, and encourages the reader to try to see what helps, rather than to rely on absolute recommendations or prescriptions.... I would recommend this book with enthusiasm to people struggling with RSD, and to those who are involved in their care in a personal and professional role."

— Dr. Amanda C de C Williams, reader in clinical health psychology
University of London, United Kingdom,
and consultant clinical psychologist

"Elena Juris's exceptionally inclusive and instructive treatise, *Positive Options,* delineates her enthusiastic, personal, 'take-charge' approach.... She blends patient accounts, physician and therapist interviews, and 'comedic moments' along with 'specific steps' bridging standard organized medicine and holistic methods. An outstanding gift of Elena's expertise is her expansive 'all-inclusive' resource list of available help in multiple areas for this condition. She has made a significant contribution."

— Marshall S. Frumin, MD,
orthopedic surgeon, Houston, Texas

"Elena Juris has put together an amazing book. It describes all types of modalities to enable the chronic sufferer to deal with the pain, discomfort, and apathy that accompany this disease. It offers tips for caregivers and suggestions on how to get appropriate treatment from physicians and other health-care professionals who really know what to do. *Positive Options* will give disheartened patients hope for better things to come and a light at the end of the dim, dark tunnel of CRPS."

— Edward Carden, MD, FRCPC, FACA, DipAAPM
director, Southern California Academic Pain Management
and Reflex Sympathetic Dystrophy Institute,
University of Southern California

"Elena bravely explores the mind–body connection and passionately articulates treating the whole person, detailing every option along the way."

— Cynthia Toussaint, founder and spokesperson
of For Grace Los Angeles, California

"Two things anyone with chronic illness needs to get better: a sense of hope and a source of support. Elena Juris provides both in this inspiring and incredibly informative book. RSD often makes people feel helpless and hopeless, but *Positive Options* changes all that. Juris provides dozens of proven ways to regain control of your health and a vast list of resources to help you do it."

— David Spero, RN, author of *The Art of Getting Well: A Five-Step Plan for Maximizing Health When You Have a Chronic Illness*

"An insightful and inspiring account for RSD sufferers and the health-care community."

— Melissa Blank, MPT, physical therapist
Baltimore, Maryland

DEDICATION

To Mom and Dad.

Positive Options
for
Complex
Regional Pain
Syndrome (CRPS)*

Self-Help and Treatment

A SECOND EDITION OF
*POSITIVE OPTIONS FOR
REFLEX SYMPATHETIC DYSTROPHY*

Elena Juris

Formerly called Reflex Sympathetic Dystrophy (RSD)

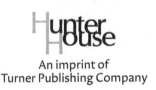

An imprint of
Turner Publishing Company

Turner Publishing Company
424 Church Street • Suite 2240 • Nashville, Tennessee 37219
445 Park Avenue • 9th Floor • New York, New York 10022
www.turnerpublishing.com

Library of Congress Cataloging-in-Publication Data
Juris, Elena.
Positive options for complex regional pain syndrome (CRPS) : self-help and
treatment / Elena Juris ; foreword by Edward Carden ; preface by
Cynthia Toussaint. — Second edition.
pages   cm
Includes bibliographical references and index.
ISBN 978-0-89793-710-8 (paperback)
ISBN 978-1-63026-613-4 (ebook)
1. Reflex sympathetic dystrophy—Popular works.   2. Reflex sympathetic
dystrophy—Treatment—Popular works.   I. Title.
RC422.R43J874 2014
616'.0472—dc23   2014020014

Project Credits
Cover Design: Jinni Fontana   Copy Editor: Amy Bauman
Book Production: John McKercher   Indexer: Jean Mooney
Developmental Editor (1st ed.):   Managing Editor: Alexandra Mummery
Kelley Blewster   Rights Coordinator: Stephanie Beard
Publisher: Kiran S. Rana

Printed and bound by Lightning Source in La Vergne, Tennessee
Manufactured in the United States of America

9 8 7 6 5 4 3 2 1   Second Edition   14 15 16 17 18

Contents

Foreword

by Dr. Edward Carden

"Hope springs eternal in the human breast."
— Alexander Pope, *An Essay on Man,* Epistle I, 1733

Is there hope for CRPS sufferers? CRPS must be the most misdiagnosed and mistreated disease in modern medicine. Because of the plethora of confusing information about the disease, the poor patient is left out in the cold. CRPS patients are often denied medical care—after being branded psychotic, shunned by their families, and left to a world of pain and suffering from which there seems to be no respite.

Elena Juris has put together an amazing book. It describes all types of modalities to enable the chronic sufferer to deal with the pain, discomfort, and apathy that accompany this disease. It offers tips for caregivers and suggestions on how to get appropriate treatment from physicians and other health-care professionals who really know what to do.

Positive Options for Complex Regional Pain Syndrome will give disheartened patients hope for better things to come and a light at the end of the dim, dark tunnel of CRPS.

— Edward Carden, MD, FRCPC, FACA, DipAAPM
director, Southern California Academic Pain Management
and Reflex Sympathetic Dystrophy Institute and retired
clinical professor, University of Southern California

Preface

by Cynthia Toussaint

"Be bold, and mighty forces will come to your aid."
— Johann Wolfgang von Goethe

Born with a fire in my belly, I've always aspired to things people told me were impossible. It was second nature for me to strive to become an accomplished ballerina and a professional actor. Fear never stood in my way, and the sublime joy of living my passion set me free. I was flying.

In 1982 a ballet injury introduced me to the world of complex regional pain syndrome (CRPS). Overnight, my life was taken from me, and for the first time fear became a part of my every moment. The fear was a darkness closing in ever so rapidly, like I was being buried one shovelful at a time. Thirteen years passed, during which I lacked a diagnosis and was repeatedly told it was all in my head. Unrelenting, spreading pain caused the fire in my belly to flicker. I was falling.

RSD brings all whom it affects to that great fork in the road: fight or flight, stand or fall. I believe we each possess the boldness to survive the great challenges of this disease and to harness "mighty forces" that will help us make the world a better place. Further, we must all find the courage to make unfamiliar choices for our own increased wellness and greater life purpose.

I dug deep to find the strength I never knew I had, and I committed to the scariest choice of all: staying—and making a difference. I redirected my passion by founding a nonprofit to heighten

RSD/CRPS awareness, and I douse my fears on a daily basis. Once again, I am flying, but this time I'm using a different set of wings.

Within the pages of *Positive Options for Complex Regional Pain Syndrome* you'll find both the knowledge to make informed choices about conventional medical treatments and the inspiration to approach alternative therapies that can complement traditional Western protocols. Elena bravely explores the mind-body connection and passionately articulates treating the whole person, detailing every option along the way. Her book promotes the concept of being an active participant in your health care; as such, it is a compelling treatise on reclaiming your life.

It has been my privilege to get to know Elena and her special brand of positive, fearless energy. Her genuine caring and compassion for the CRPS community resonates deeply within me, and I reflect fondly upon the conversations we've had—often speaking over one another with enthusiasm about the all-embracing, holistic approach of her book. I admire and applaud her strength and vision to step away from the familiar trend, leaving "safe" behind.

I encourage each of us with CRPS, along with our loved ones and caregivers, to follow Elena's affirming example of stepping out of the box and taking strident actions to make the world aware of CRPS, creating a tapestry of broader support and finer understanding of this condition. Let us turn our backs on fear and approach each day with the courage to do the impossible; that's how hope stays alive and fires remain stoked.

Be bold. With boldness, the seemingly insurmountable and the defiantly inconceivable melt away to a tableau of new lands charted, of sky-high mountains scaled.

— Cynthia Toussaint
Founder and spokesperson, For Grace,
and author, *Battle for Grace*

Acknowledgments

So many thanks to Dr. Bleecker for catching me right before I hit rock bottom, to Sheri for carrying me back up, to Sam for always believing in me, and to Kim (wifie) for keeping me sane and encouraged (and well brushed!). To Aunt Helen for her soothing talks, along with Uncle Phil and Jeremy for hosting a nurturing island in New York. To Jennifer for her late-night chats, reminding me that I still had the power to be funny. To Arpi for her companionship at such a difficult time, and to Dominique for her thoughtful letters pushing me to think outside of my walls. To Jesse and Jessica for their open visiting hours. And to the five Jacobs' "Badonkadonks" for their amazing love and generosity: I have made their friendships my own religion.

I'm thankful to all the friends and family I feel I got to know better through this experience—and to the strangers who offered so much random kindness. I thank everyone in the RSD/pain community who has shared his or her knowledge and stories with me, and the readers who have convinced me this past decade that this book helped them. To Marci, Janelle, and Christine for helping make the Center for Occupational and Environmental Neurology (COEN) a peaceful, welcoming place to come to, and to the folks at Hand N Hand for making a big transition so seamless. To Hunter House, for giving this book a chance and providing an excellent partner through Alex. Finally, to Mom, Dad, and Joel for opening their doors and tolerating a temperamental adult daughter or stepdaughter in their midst. To Dad for his extended company, endless diversions, and late-night mangoes. And to Mom: Thanks for always letting me feel that someone understood every rainbow of pain and emotion through every step, every moment. I love you.

A lot has changed since I wrote the first edition of this book. In this second edition, I'd like to thank my husband, Kristan, my "sherpa," who endures my sometimes bottomless expressions of frustration and grief when pain tests my spirit; your humor at dark times is a treasure. I am also grateful to Navi Kaur for her research assistance in this updated edition, and the overseas contributions of Rukmini Chatterjee. Finally, my move to Washington, DC, a decade ago reaped many blessings beyond mobility and a new career path: It led to a community of supportive old and new friends who have left a lifelong impression of sweetness on these years of rebuilding my life; you know who you are, and I am blessed to have you in it.

Important Note

The material in this book is intended to provide a review of resources and information related to complex regional pain syndrome types 1 and 2 (formerly called reflex sympathetic dystrophy and causalgia, respectively). Every effort has been made to provide accurate and dependable information. However, professionals in the field may have differing opinions, and change is always taking place. Any of the treatments described herein should be undertaken only under the guidance of a licensed health-care practitioner. The author, editors, and publishers cannot be held responsible for any error, omission, professional disagreement, outdated material, or adverse outcomes that derive from use of any of the treatments or information resources in this book, either in a program of self-care or under the care of a licensed practitioner.

Introduction

If you're holding this book open with your feet or a bookstand because it hurts too much to use your hands, you're in the right place.

Maybe you're in a wheelchair because pain in your leg prevents you from walking. If so, stay right where you are, and read on. You also belong here.

For the rest of you: If you are awed or devastated by the fact that burning pain has apparently commandeered the emotional life of your loved one and you want to help, please join us.

If you think you're suffering alone with complex regional pain syndrome (CRPS), I'm writing this book to prove otherwise. Even though the hypersensitized nerve condition (historically known as reflex sympathetic dystrophy, or RSD) is considered mysterious and underdiagnosed, it is now estimated that fifty thousand new cases appear in the United States each year. Suspected to be a dysfunctional reaction to minor bodily trauma ranging from a minor cut or sprained ankle to carpal tunnel surgery, it can happen to anyone at any time. Most disastrously, the challenge within the medical community to ensure an accurate diagnosis, deliver effective treatment, and have access to relevant research outcomes often leaves patients completely lost as a cloud of debate rages around them—at the very moment when they most need help.

I am writing as a CRPS/RSD survivor rather than as a doctor. I have conducted an extensive amount of research into CRPS, and in this book I have provided in-depth information on the condition, its various features, and the range of methods available to treat it. Because of the intense nature of CRPS pain, you will discover you have quite a few things to learn about living with the condition after you've been diagnosed and have started your medical treatment. Losing the carefree use of a hand, an arm, a leg, or more; monitoring the minute-by-minute burning pain; and witnessing the effects of your condition on your family, friends, career, and financial situation are burdens you must bear outside of the doctor's office. My aim in writing this book is to provide a guide for inspiration amid those challenges.

My Experience with CRPS

Over the course of one year, I became an invalid with CRPS in both arms and then was tenderly coaxed back into being an upright person who has learned to live with and manage her condition. Throughout the ordeal, I was forced to leave my rising career at age twenty-six, move back home with my parents, and watch a myriad of friends and family help me do everything from showering to brushing my teeth. I found myself unable to concentrate, cook, clean, comb my hair, or drive a car, and I spent many sleepless, frantic nights struggling to maintain my cool as burning pain laid siege to my arms. By day, I scoured every available resource for information on CRPS—and was terrified by the overwhelming clinical information and abundant horror stories that I found in place of encouragement. By night, I surprised myself by contemplating hand amputations or suicide to simply end the pain.

To regain control over my terrified and grieving self, I avoided sources of information on CRPS that reminded me negatively of my mysterious disease, and instead reached elsewhere as well as inward for ammunition with which to combat my moment-to-moment despair. I learned that one of the most important things I could do was stay calm. I received extensive support throughout this process—something that so few patients find amidst the blur of constant acute pain, compounding loss, and labyrinthine debates with doctors and insurance carriers. Selected medical experts, family, and close friends carried me through the experience with encouragement and faith. That's not to say that my first chance at diagnosis wasn't overlooked at an internationally renowned U.S. hospital, that I don't have a number of negative medical office experiences to share, or that my closest friends and family provided exactly the support I needed without struggle. Rather, I will focus on what *did* work during this ordeal. For that, I am grateful.

I found a neurologist and occupational therapist who spent the time to explain to me the crucial interaction in CRPS between mind, body, and spirit. Acupuncture and other complementary therapies greatly aided my healing and pain management. I explored my own means of distracting and expanding my mind and dug deep enough to find the sense of humor and playful spirit that I had all but forgotten. I had to look at myself as someone forever changed, and—here's the hard part—I had to learn to be at peace with my new life paradigm, even if I also knew that better treatments for CRPS always remain on the horizon. Otherwise, as much as I wanted to repeat "CRPS has destroyed my life" over and over again, I would have been the one suffering from recycled anger and grief by focusing on the negative.

My journey to reclaim certain abilities from my former life still continues, but the constant burning siege has stopped. With drug therapy, acupuncture, occupational therapy, manual therapy, and lifestyle modifications, I'm in control of my body once again. Since the time this book was originally published a decade ago, I had a relapse that lasted seven months. Yet, my life is *again* active and back in my hands and has been a story of remission for at least seven years: I re-entered the workforce years ago, eventually rebuilding my career with the aid of assistive technology. I got married. I pursue selected hobbies in a limited fashion, and I am carefully back in the gym. While my nervous system has since stabilized, I still learn new clues every day about keeping a close, yet forgiving, dialogue with my body.

Support Is Available

One element held true throughout this entire experience: Support was available to me if I knew where to look for it. And, boy, did I look! This is the knowledge I want to share with you. In *Positive Options for Complex Regional Pain Syndrome (CRPS)* you'll find a wealth of tips on how to modify your lifestyle so you can better manage your condition and feel more empowered. You'll find two interviews with practitioners that offer insights that every patient should know. You'll find a discussion of complementary therapies that you can try out and customize for your own treatment needs. You'll find a list of "dynamite distractions" that can refresh your mind and help you rediscover your light, creative, and silly sides for when you just need to take your mind off the illness. You'll find a chapter addressed to loved ones that provides advice and support to them in their difficult roles as encouragers and caregivers. You'll find information on how everyone can help to increase CRPS/RSD awareness, and in the back of the book, you'll find an extensive list of resources that will help you begin to implement all of these suggestions.

CRPS can be an isolating condition, not only because so few people understand it, but also because patients too often remain isolated from other patients' triumphs. It's important for you to know that the possibility of recovering from your lowest place does exist. What better way to testify to this fact than through the direct words of CRPS patients and survivors? Scattered throughout the book, you'll find encouraging stories of healing and learning from actual CRPS patients. The contributors represent many ages, have suffered the gamut of symptoms, and have experienced various degrees of improvement. All of them embody strength of will, an open mind, and generosity in sharing their stories. Each contributor has embraced an individualized approach to dealing with CRPS, and each one offers something that too few CRPS patients have easy access to: real-life hope.

You can keep this book on your nightstand as an inspirational pick-me-up or use it as a reference guide to treatments and helpful products or services. Thumb through the book for guidance in preparing to see a new doctor or explore the insights imparted by the medical professionals interviewed within. Consider keeping the book open to certain pages conveniently listing activities that can be gentle, accessible, and bring you instant gratification. Mark some text that uniquely speaks to you about reframing your life situation, and read those lines daily, if not hourly. If you're a caregiver, review the chapter devoted to your unique challenges and use it to find support for yourself. Whether you're a CRPS patient or caregiver, consider this book a nurturing companion that reminds you of the *positive* options available to you and your family for dealing with the complex syndrome known as CRPS. Learning about these options now can save you essential time by preventing you from having to discover them at random later.

Please be optimistic and believe that your life will get better. CRPS *can* go into remission—or in many cases it can at least improve enough to be managed within a full and vibrant life. Awareness of and research into this condition have improved in past years. The most important things you can bring to the effort are a belief in your own rich spirit and resourcefulness. Maintain affirmative thoughts; they can buffer your response to pain by subduing the anxiety that only further excites your nervous system. Learn what triggers a flare-up of your illness and have faith in your ability to intercept and break this excruciating cycle. With practice, you can regain more control. Doing so, however, will take time. And patience. It is all about baby steps. So let's take our first few.

What Is CRPS?

CRPS is...gritting my teeth as I feel the excruciating crunch of every water droplet between my burning fingers after struggling through a shower. CRPS is...suffering the humiliation of waiting all day until someone ties my shoes and opens the front door for me. CRPS is...deadly cold hands that cannot bear the touch of a soothing hand to warm them. CRPS is...anxiety, fear, and frustration, alienation, desperation, and immense loss. It is navigating a medical community that is insufficiently informed and regularly fails at diagnosing this serious pain condition, thus endangering patients suffering with it.

But wait: There is also good news. CRPS also involves being detected and embraced by the certain dedicated health professionals who slowly educated and nursed me back to life. And finally, CRPS involves healing.

This has been my experience, with full knowledge that each person's story is a unique shape in the CRPS mosaic. Yet for all the many ways that CRPS assaults its sufferers, so too is there a way to heal various facets of your life that have been turned upside down by this mysterious and complex condition. CRPS experts have confirmed that the most comprehensive treatment of CRPS must integrate psychological support with medical and complementary care for optimal results. As a result, the therapeutic directions you can take in CRPS management are plentiful.

This book offers restorative methods for the newly diagnosed and the old-timer alike. Whether it be a new treatment, an adaptation in daily activity, a daring practice in comforting your soul, a deeper level of understanding between you and your loved ones, a blissful distraction, or a different way of looking at yourself, you'll find them all here. When the same old bursts of burning pain still shock and surprise you, or panicked doubts and questions rage through your mind in the middle of the night, you can reach for this book as an inspirational reminder of therapeutic tricks—or a source of new learning. As you embark on your own search for information about your condition, I offer this book as a companion to your life and your personal episode with CRPS.

The first step in making peace with CRPS is to understand it. Though a simple feat in the case of many diseases, knowing how and why your pain occurs in CRPS presents unique challenges to you and your doctor. Even the name can be a source of confusion: Since 1993 complex regional pain syndrome (type 1) has been the descriptive new name for what was previously known as (and sometimes still is) reflex sympathetic dystrophy (RSD). In other parts of the world, different names for this same condition exist: posttraumatic dystrophy, algodystrophy, minor causalgia, algoneurodystrophy, shoulder-hand syndrome, and Sudeck's atrophy. Complex regional pain syndrome (type 2), which is far less common and involves a major precipitating nerve trauma, has been previously known as causalgia; however, despite this distinction in causation, CRPS type 1 and 2 symptoms and general treatment responses evidently tend to be the same. To be most inclusive of both the old and the new medical terminology, I will use *CRPS* within this book, but I occasionally include the old name, if appropriate; for example, major advocacy organizations have retained their traditional names for the disorder.

A phenomenon that existed well before it was named, CRPS is a debilitating, multisystem condition characterized by severe burning pain, pathological changes in bone and skin, excessive sweating, tissue swelling, and extreme sensitivity to touch. In roughly 65 percent of CRPS cases, a mere soft-tissue injury, such as a sprained ankle, progresses into the condition. Fractures, surgeries, spinal cord disorders, injections, infections, and repetitive strain injuries, such as carpal tunnel syndrome, also can precipitate CRPS. Eight percent of people with a Colles fracture develop CRPS, and upper extremities are twice as likely to be affected as lower limbs. It is estimated that 2 to 5 percent of injuries affecting peripheral nerves can develop into CRPS, and 12 to 20 percent of individuals paralyzed on one side of the body develop the condition. In some cases, a particular cause of CRPS is never found; in others, the condition developed in response to something as minor as a spider bite or a needle stick. It is estimated that fifty-thousand new CRPS (type 1) cases occur annually in the United States, and a Dutch population study suggested that 40.4 females and 11. 9 males develop the condition among 100,000 person-years at risk.

Features of CRPS

CRPS symptoms can manifest themselves in many different forms, but the signature feature—and heartbreak—of CRPS is severe, unrelenting pain that far exceeds the expected discomfort of the initial injury. The pain can be deep, burning, and constant, spreading beyond the area of injury. Sharp jabs of pain *(paroxysmal disesthesias* and *lancinating pains),* aching pain, electrical sensations, and small muscle spasms can also plague the affected region. Additionally, a condition called *allodynia* can commonly occur, which makes any stimulation of the affected area an agonizing experience, even if it is a light breeze or soft touch that normally would not cause any pain at all.

While an individual can develop CRPS anywhere in the body, it usually begins in one or more extremities, initially distributing itself along the hand or foot in what is called a "glove and stocking" pattern. Uniquely affecting the nerves, skin, blood vessels, bones, and muscles, the condition presents overlapping stages of severity and progresses at a different pace in each person. At its onset, the skin of the affected regions can first become warm and shiny, swollen, and reveal a reddish, bluish, or mottled white color. Sweating abnormalities can also take place, usually in the form of *hyperhidrosis,* or increased sweating. Joints can become stiff, limiting movement and causing muscle atrophy and further pain.

Why do these particular changes occur? Doctors and researchers are still in the process of pinpointing and agreeing upon exactly why, but they do know that a dysfunction in the body's natural healing process is taking place. Normally, when body tissue is injured, it releases chemicals called *cytokines,* which both initiate the nerve transmission of warning pain signals and attract restorative blood and tissue cells to the damaged area. Fluid also leaks from the damaged blood vessels, causing swelling, or *edema,* if the veins are unable to remove the excess liquid. As blood cleanses and pumps through the injured tissue, the tissue normally heals and edema disappears. However, with CRPS, an interruption in this natural process prevents healing, often causing constant inflammation. A disruption in normal circulation occurs as well, further obstructing healing by causing dilation of arteries, which leads to more fluid leakage into affected tissues.

Meanwhile, contraction of blood vessels, or *vasoconstriction,* also occurs intermittently, leaving veins unable to remove unhealthy nonprotein fluid from tissues. As a result, swelling continues much longer than normal and progressively causes stiffness and limited mobility in an ever-perpetuating loop. This downward spiral constantly irritates pain-causing nerve endings, or *nociceptors,* which makes it increasingly painful for patients to move the affected area.

CRPS's interference with circulation via autonomic dysregulation can cause the extremities to feel chronically cold or hot, causing some cases to be termed "cold CRPS" or "hot CRPS." Additionally, if blood vessels become constricted, skin discoloration can occur, and skin, tendons, ligaments, and bones may fail to receive their proper nutrients. The skin can become cold and blue, and nails can begin to grow at an accelerated rate. Despite wishful thinking, the pain of this condition does not simply burn itself out over time without treatment.

Advanced CRPS

Traditionally, experts have broken the syndrome into three or four stages of progression, with most patients never progressing to stage four. However, since symptoms can be found in various stages, and because what we know about the disease is still changing, these stages are not clearly defined and merely serve as fluid guidelines for doctors. (For example, CRPS in my hands never showed remarkable swelling; instead, my hands directly entered a cold, sweating state with burning, perfuse allodynia and early contractures.) It is often found, however, that if CRPS progresses or continues untreated, the pain and limited mobility of joints intensifies, and ligaments and tendons can contract. Osteoporosis can occur and becomes diffuse in affected bones. As affected muscles waste away, continued inactivity of the involved limb or region perpetuates the hypersensitivity and pain of CRPS. Other complications of advanced and chronic CRPS can include systemic effects, from memory disturbances and motor impairment, to dermatological, urological, gastrointestinal, adrenal, cardiac, and respiratory involvement.

Patients may not experience the symptoms in the same order or pattern, and not all patients experience all of the symptoms. For an overview on these evolving stages, visit http://www.rsdhope.org /crps-stages.html; the site continues to be updated. Remember:

Although CRPS can be a progressive disorder, it does not advance in all cases. The key to a positive prognosis is prompt diagnosis and treatment.

What Causes CRPS?

Theories about CRPS and its origins continue to evolve. Originally CRPS was believed to be the result of a dysfunction of the sympathetic nervous system, which is the system in charge of regulating body temperature, sensory reception, pulse, respiration, blood pressure (dilation and constriction of blood vessels), and the part of the immune system that stabilizes inflammation. The sympathetic nervous system is composed of the nerves that control the autonomic or "self-ruling" body functions—those over which you do not have voluntary control. On many fronts, the sympathetic nervous system's role in CRPS makes sense to doctors, as it controls the start and stop of the fight-or-flight survival response you have in response to any emergency, including injuries and pain. The original name for CRPS type 1, *reflex sympathetic dystrophy,* reflected this theory.

However, evidence shows that pain in CRPS is not always sympathetically maintained; in other words, patients can experience pain that is independent of the sympathetic nervous system. More recently, CRPS has been recognized as a disease of the broader central nervous system. Studies have shown that in the brain's somatosensory cortex, the area corresponding to a patient's affected limb actually shrinks; this gray matter shrinkage correlates to pain and duration changes in CRPS patients. The cause and chronic nature of CRPS may be blamed on the interrelated dysfunction of both the nervous system and the immune system. Evidence that the condition can become "imprinted" in the central nervous system can be shown through symptoms such as physiological tremor, which is caused by central changes in approximately 50 percent of patients.

Certain receptor sites on nerves in the spinal cord—the ones that process and transmit pain information to the brain—can become chronically overstimulated. After an initial traumatic injury, such chronic overstimulation can lead to CRPS. Think of it in terms of how you try to remember something. You keep repeating the information until your brain cells finally "get it" and memorize the lesson. Certain cells in the spinal cord also seem to have an ability to remember certain types of stimulation. It may be a very crude form of memory, but nevertheless, it is a form of memory. In CRPS, your reaction to pain, experience of pain, response to external danger, and ability to heal tissue damage and maintain a functional balance among systems are all compromised, throwing off the complex system of checks and balances that your body normally maintains. The result is pain, which in itself causes more pain by the havoc it wreaks on your nervous and immune systems. Set rolling in a constantly reactive state, the sympathetic and central nervous systems are left abnormally excited or sensitive, their neurons spastically firing pain signals at the smallest stimulation—or even without any stimulation at all.

This loss of equilibrium, or loss of *homeostasis,* is not only physical. Also affected is the limbic system, the part of the central nervous system that resides in the cerebral cortex of the brain and largely governs emotions, pleasure, and pain cognition. It is responsible for producing *endorphins,* hormones that provide feelings of euphoria and pain relief, and enhance sleep. Within the cycle of constant neuropathic pain, inflammation in the limbic system causes intense anxiety, agitation, insomnia, depression, memory disturbances, poor concentration, and sometimes panic attacks in a majority of CRPS patients. Recent theories suggest that the effects of this pattern over time can actually become permanently set in the brain and, in addition to changes in the spinal cord, account for the various other physical and mental complications that CRPS patients can experience. Research continues to examine the autonomic dysfunction, neurogenic inflammation, and neuroplastic central nervous system changes that all play a part in the condition's pathophysiology.

The CRPS Cycle

Although the specific, comprehensive mechanisms of CRPS are still being delineated, the simplified diagram in Figure 1 represents a very basic spiral of hyperexcitability and pain that can start to help you to picture the dysfunction.

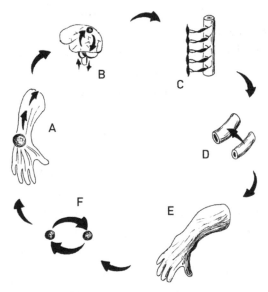

FIGURE 1. The CRPS cycle. A) Injury to arm and hands starts the cycle; B) original injury initiates a pain impulse carried by sensory nerves to the central nervous system; C) the pain impulse in turn triggers an impulse in the sympathetic nervous system that returns to the original site of injury; D) the sympathetic impulse triggers the inflammatory response causing the vessel to spasm, leading to swelling and increased pain; E) resulting condition with burning extremity pain, red mottling of the skin; F) the pain triggers another response, establishing a cycle of pain and swelling.

Understanding this loss of internal homeostasis will help you imagine the range and methods of treatments used to treat your condition, and the theories behind the treatments will help you understand how you can enhance your own treatment.

Why You?

Why these dysfunctions originally take place is still largely unknown. There are, however, some suspected reasons for why one person develops CRPS and another person doesn't. Some experts suggest that instigators can include the disuse of an affected body part for an extended time (e.g., cast, brace, bed rest, or overprotection) or the repetitive application of ice to an injury, interfering with circulation to that area. The chance of developing CRPS may increase with hereditary factors, with family history of CRPS showing more involvement of multiple affected limbs than sporadic cases. While a notable family history showed in 6 to 15 percent of cases in some studies, the inheritance pattern is not yet clear, or may involve interactions among multiple genes. Females between the ages of forty and sixty develop the condition most frequently. In fact, between two thirds and three quarters of adult CRPS patients are women; even 90 percent of reported pediatric cases involve eight- to sixteen-year-old girls.

Certain surgeries or injuries may create higher risks for CRPS development as well, such as back and arthroscopic knee surgery. Invasive procedures to treat nerve entrapments such as carpal tunnel syndrome, tarsal tunnel syndrome, or thoracic outlet syndrome can also aggravate already existing inflammation and nerve pain, inviting CRPS to develop. In a study of CRPS patients with a fractured bone, intra-articular fractures, ankle fractures, and dislocations were the most frequent culprits. Blast injuries seen in wartime can also pose a risk; during the years of U.S. engagement in Iraq and Afghanistan, hundreds of new CRPS cases were reported to the U.S. Department of Veterans Affairs. Some say that having extra stress in your life at the time of initial injury can also be a risk factor.

Hopefully, with increased awareness of CRPS, those with injuries or those undergoing procedures with higher risk of developing CRPS can be more carefully treated to prevent or minimize the syndrome in the future. Under the care of informed medical professionals, early mobilization of the extremities after an injury or stroke could aid prevention. Additional prophylactic measures, such as the administration of vitamin C to prevent toxic radical damage after a fracture, have shown promise. In one such study of 127 wrist-fracture patients, the incidence of CRPS was reduced to 7 percent of the patients receiving 500 milligrams (mg) of vitamin C daily, as opposed to 22 percent in patients receiving a placebo.

In addition, increased awareness in the medical community can also reduce the spread of CRPS in diagnosed patients who must undergo additional surgeries. Receiving a nerve block in the affected area during surgery can help, as can adding ketamine to the anesthesia of some CRPS patients undergoing surgeries. In one study of patients in remission who had to undergo surgery on their originally affected arm, IV regional anesthesia with combined lidocaine and clonidine made an extraordinary impact on reducing the recurrence of CRPS in that arm.

Diagnosis

Early diagnosis is crucial in providing the most optimal outcome for CRPS recovery. Yet because there is no single external test for CRPS, diagnosis remains a sticky subject for patients, doctors, and insurance carriers. A doctor's clinical diagnosis is key to effective RSD/CRPS intervention. Unfortunately, many doctors remain unaware of CRPS or simply do not consider it until patients have passed through months or even years of excruciating pain and damage. Sometimes, CRPS is mistakenly diagnosed as thromboembolistic disease or a rheumatic disease. (I, personally, was sent to a rheumatologist who could not explain why I suddenly felt like my palms were on fire.) It is not unusual for patients to have visited numerous doctors before being diagnosed and to have been accused of imagining the pain before the severity of the condition is realized. Such experiences add to the toxic role stress plays in a patient's snowballing pain. To find out how you can help change this situation, read Chapter 9 for a discussion of several simple ways you can encourage awareness of CRPS in the medical community and among the general population.

Diagnostic Tests

A promising and sensitive diagnostic tool is thermal imaging, or infrared *thermography*. Thermal imaging painlessly provides a picture of the temperature(s) of different parts of the body. Often used to check for vascular insufficiency or pulled muscles, the test can identify "hot" CRPS regions and "cold" CRPS regions by revealing heat differentials. Skin temperature asymmetries between the affected and opposite limb of roughly around 36° Fahrenheit (2° Celsius), combined with patient history and symptoms, provide reliable data for a clinician to make a diagnosis. In cases that are more difficult to identify, an autonomic stress test is sometimes performed. This test might require that you step into a bucket of cold water while the temperature of both hands is monitored by thermal imaging. If one hand turns cold (as expected) and the other becomes hotter, the degree of difference in temperature is revealed and offers clues to the dysfunction of your autonomic nervous system. Once treatment starts, thermal imaging can also track your progress.

Imaging equipment is expensive, and doctors must complete an extensive training course in order to be properly certified to use it. These factors significantly limit the widespread use of thermal imaging. In addition, some doctors dismiss the validity of the thermography test. However, many workers' compensation policies and private insurance carriers pay for the test to be conducted. Its benefits are obvious not only for patients and doctors but also for insurance purposes, because the test can show if a patient is indeed exaggerating his or her pain.

Drawbacks still exist, however. Thermography can reveal reduced blood flow to an area, but it's important to note that peripheral nerve entrapments can cause similar vascular insufficiency. To track down a professional who is qualified to conduct the test, check with the American Academy of Medical Infrared Imaging (see the Resources section). The doctor does not have to be the same doctor with whom you pursue treatment.

Doctors may resort to other various tools, such as bone scans or a positive response to a sympathetic nerve block treatment, to confirm the presence of CRPS. Unfortunately, not every patient's bone scan reveals bone wasting; a patient must usually enter a more advanced stage of CRPS damage in order to reveal evidence of bone wasting. Additionally, treating a patient by using sympathetic nerve blocks in order to retroactively diagnose and prove that she has the condition is often a less-than-satisfactory protocol for doctors. Moreover, not every case of CRPS features sympathetically maintained pain, so not every CRPS patient responds to such treatment.

Doctors might also use other tests, such as nerve conduction studies, magnetic resonance imaging (MRI), X rays, and electromyography (EMG), to investigate other sources of pain. However, it is important to note that conditions revealed by such tests, such as carpal tunnel syndrome, can in fact develop into CRPS and can coexist with CRPS. (I personally developed CRPS as a result of a poorly treated repetitive strain injury in my wrist.) This leaves a major challenge for the medical community, once a diagnosis is made: integratively managing CRPS and comorbid conditions.

Clinical Diagnosis

A doctor's hands-on clinical skills must be relied on to piece together an accurate diagnosis, paying careful attention to a patient's history leading up to the pain. Time is of the essence. While it is important to rule out other potential conditions and ensure a different diagnosis from radiculopathy or nerve entrapments, full attention should be paid to the symptoms at hand. In addition to listening to the patient's story and examining the area affected, a simple test that a doctor can conduct during clinical evaluation is called the Hendler alcohol drop and swipe test. This test involves testing the patient's thermal and mechanical allodynia by evaluating his or her response to the sensation of cold alcohol on the skin (thermal) and of a cotton swab stroking the skin (mechanical).

Diagnostic Criteria

Due to the hard work of activists, the Social Security Administration passed official diagnostic criteria for recognizing CRPS in October 2003. Symptoms considered for a diagnosis include pain (severe, burning, constant, deep, sharp, shooting, electrical, or crushing) that is well beyond what is normal for the inciting event, that impairs mobility, and that occurs along with one or more of the following:

- autonomic instability, seen in the form of skin changes (dry, shiny, scaly; mottled, red, or blue; coarse hair growth or thinning; faster or slower nail growth; excessive or decreased sweating; heightened warmth or coolness)
- swelling (pitted or hard)
- movement disorders (diminished mobility; stiffness, spasms, tremors; dystonia, as in drawing up of the hands or toes)
- osteoporosis
- spreading of symptoms (traveling up the extremity, to the opposite limb, or elsewhere)

It is important to remember that not every CRPS patient will reveal all the "classic" symptoms. For example, I did not experience any swelling whatsoever. Furthermore, while the sweating and scaliness in my hands resolved within months, a drawing up of my fingers into what I called "monkey hand" came on slowly and persisted intermittently for two years.

Ultimately a doctor may make a diagnosis of one of the following:

* CRPS type 1, formerly known as RSD, which involves minor trauma or injury
* CRPS type 2, formally known as causalgia, which involves injury to a major nerve (as in gunshot or shrapnel injuries)

Essentially, symptoms and treatment overlap for both types of CRPS.

In 2007 the International Association for the Study of Pain (IASP) released updated diagnostic criteria for RSD/CRPS. Unfortunately some debate surrounds its lack of specificity and its propensity to lead to overdiagnosis.

Brenda's story highlights some of the challenges a patient can face when trying to get an accurate diagnosis for this confounding syndrome.

Brenda's Story

Twenty-four hours after bunion surgery, I had symptoms of CRPS. I experienced constant burning pain from my ankle to the back of my knee for six weeks, then it began to move up my leg. All the skin peeled off my left foot. I had stiff joints (which I thought were due to my not moving around enough), severe spasms in my foot lasting maybe fifteen to thirty seconds, and "Charlie horse" cramps. I couldn't sleep well at night. Maybe I'd sleep for three hours and then I'd have to take painkillers, and then it would take another hour to get back to sleep. This got even worse as time went on. Then a new symptom set in that I didn't recognize—I could feel the line of the nerve all the way up to my hip. Six weeks after surgery, on a bright morning in January 2001, I woke up with the burning pain on one side of my face! Within two weeks, it covered 90 percent of my body.

I was started on aggressive physical therapy three weeks post-op. My primary doctor thought it was only tendonitis; however, I later saw the physical therapist's notes, which clearly stated "early RSD." My doctor never acknowledged this opinion. I've worked in the medical field myself, so I want to tell everyone who thinks they have RSD that they need to recognize there are different viewpoints about the syndrome, just like there are for fibromyalgia and other conditions. My MD would not refer me willingly to a pain-management doctor, but she did refer me quickly to a rehabilitation MD. He confirmed the diagnosis of RSD. I was also eventually referred to a neurologist.

I kept a journal of my symptoms for the first four months because my sister, who is in the medical field, suggested it might help my doctors narrow down what my problem was. The spreading of pain from the original areas continued for six weeks. It covered all of my body except my right hand, and in some parts it seemed to be more comprehensive than in others. For one week, the only comfortable position for me was standing. I experienced swelling that felt like a band around my chest, severe headaches, and sensitivity to sound—such that I could not have music on, and even the turn signal in the car was too loud. During the day, I frequently had stabbing pains throughout my leg, foot, and pelvis.

From July to November 2002 the neurologist told me that there was "no such thing as RSD or CRPS." I told him he could call it anything he wanted, "just don't call me crazy." He wanted to call it neuralgia, unspecified. He suspected multiple sclerosis (MS), but he had to rule out a host of other things. It was a very long four months before the results of the spinal tests were in. Honestly, I believe the only way I lasted four months believing I could have both CRPS *and* MS was by holding on to my faith in God and my belief that He would see me through.

I went to the Cleveland Clinic for a second opinion. The staff felt they could easily rule out MS. Meanwhile, my neurologist felt I was jumping into hot water by "looking" for this diagnosis. He would have rather listed me as "ruled out MS" for years than to diagnose me with RSD/CRPS.

I've had RSD now for twenty-one months and probably have been in "remission" since May 2003. However, I define remission as simply having my condition controlled by medications. So it all depends on how you define remission!

Looking back, I can offer the following advice to others: I minimized how much pain I was in. If you can't sleep more than four hours at a time, the doctor needs to prescribe something else—perhaps not a pain med, but definitely a sleep med at night. Also, when you're getting referred to a specialist, ask your primary doctor to have his or her office call to make an appointment for you ASAP; otherwise it can take a long time. There was a two-month wait to get in to see my pain-management specialist! If your doctor won't help, then drive to the next city to get help sooner.

I don't think neurologists are trained in the same way as pain-management doctors are. Just recognize that their training is different and try to not let them frustrate you. I have heard of only one case that was originally considered RSD that turned out to be MS. MS can be very painful, and some cases can be very similar to RSD, but MS usually isn't related to an injury, and it usually doesn't have a sudden onset like RSD/CRPS. The neurologist will prescribe the testing you may need to rule out some things, so be polite but don't negate your own experiences.

Finding a Doctor

As Brenda's story shows, "CRPS/RSD experts" run the gamut in medical disciplines, from anesthesiologists to neurologists to orthopedic surgeons, and so on. As a result, more than one particular type of doctor can demonstrate an interest and willingness to serve as your advocate. Various professionals, for reasons of personal experience or by chance of clinical contact with many CRPS patients, have developed significant experience in identifying and working with CRPS patients through the long haul. If the most renowned orthopedic surgeon in your area does not treat you and your case with respect, it is okay to seek a second opinion—or a third—until you find someone who is ready to address your pain.

In my experience, if an orthopedist fails to offer insights, try a neurologist or a pain management specialist in your area. People are out there who are familiar with the type of symptoms you are describing! Call the office and ask if the doctors have treated RSD/CRPS; it is worth seeking them out. Moreover, another type of doctor—such as a physiatrist (who specializes in physical rehabilitation)—might be well suited to help you integrate rehabilitative care and adapt to a new lifestyle once your initial treatment is on track.

An excellent way to guide your search is to find a practitioner who is certified in pain medicine or pain management/anesthesiology. These are professionals (such as neurologists and anesthesiologists) officially certified by the American Board of Pain Medicine after significant additional training (not just occasional courses or seminars). They can serve as your primary health-care provider or serve as a close counselor to another professional treating you.

In addition to asking around about someone who your friends, family, or colleagues recommend for addressing pain, you can check with your local chapter of the American Academy of Pain Medicine, American Pain Society, or American Chronic Pain Association. Is your doctor a member of the International Association for the Study of Pain? Your state or county medical society and the American Board of Medical Specialties can verify a doctor's credentials. Also, you can check the following websites for specific doctor listings in your area—some including patient feedback.

www.healthgrades.com

www.findadoc.com

The Reflex Sympathetic Dystrophy Syndrome Association of America is a resource for patients seeking experienced pain doctors in their state. Finally, another alternative is to check online for a doctor who has published papers on your symptoms or on CRPS. Since this doctor has demonstrated a passion for studying the condition, she or he may be someone who can help you or who can recommend a colleague in your area.

You and Your Doctor

It cannot be emphasized enough how important the doctor-patient relationship is in managing and potentially healing CRPS. Your doctor's willingness to listen and, if necessary, to research and learn more about treating you is critically important. Your doctor needs to be willing in advance to create and discuss a strategy of options, or a *treatment protocol,* to serve specific goals; realizing that your doctor is haphazardly choosing random treatments can detrimentally increase anxiety about your future and your doctor's competence.

Ask your doctor what portion of his practice is devoted to chronic pain patients, what treatment options he is willing to explore with pain patients, and if he is a member of any pain-management association. What is her philosophy towards CRPS pain management? What about complementary treatment? Does she attend and participate in pain conferences?

You need to feel a rapport with your doctor and to sense that he or she trusts and *believes* you. This mutual trust can be one of the strongest links in your treatment. Finally, if you have just been diagnosed with CRPS, your doctor needs to be *frequently available to you,* at least in the beginning, as time is of the essence in intensively treating the condition. Find out how long it would take to get an appointment in an emergency and also find out what your doctor does in case of after-hours emergencies. For more information on locating a doctor, check the Resources section in the back of the book. Partners Against Pain offers downloadable resources for tracking and discussing your pain with your doctor: www.partnersagainstpain.com.

Some CRPS patients do manage their own treatment, rather than relying on a single doctor as case manager. It can be a frustrating reality best faced by learning as much as possible about the condition and fearlessly pursuing the resources out there. Gather your advocates and your experts, depending on what underlying injury or procedure may have initially sparked the CRPS. For Kathleen, although she initially searched for a doctor who could oversee her care, being forced to manage her own recovery turned out to have hidden benefits.

K athleen's Story

Two years ago I was hobbling about my workplace a month following routine foot surgery. My colleagues shared my distress about the ice-cold feel and blue color of my foot as well as my ankle that was swollen to the size of my knee. The pain felt like a thousand tiny paper cuts, awash with ammonia and reopening with every step. Tears would come and go at work as I was distracted by the relentless, burning pain. Sleep was elusive, and shopping, cooking, and cleaning for my eight- and ten-year-olds was exhausting. I felt like the choo-choo with square wheels on the Island of Misfit Toys who didn't hope for round wheels but only that Santa would find a child who would want it. I also found it hard to imagine my foot would roll smoothly again. It was enough just to endure another day.

My podiatrist recognized the classic symptoms of RSD/CRPS four weeks following surgery, and he initiated physical therapy that same day. Two months later, I ran out of insurance and was far from "over it." I kept doing the therapy routine at home but was lonely and frightened. I wasn't getting far in my hopes to drive with my right foot and walk without a limp, much less play catch with my son or soccer with my daughter.

A month after working on my own, I discovered a professor at the University of Puget Sound, where I work. Dr. Roger Allen taught neuroanatomy in the Doctor of Physical Therapy program at the university and specialized in treatment of CRPS. I learned from him that the "C" in CRPS partly meant that no one really understood the cause of this condition, and thus the healing process would be equally challenging. What might work for another, might not for me. In early conversations, he stressed the importance of a multidisciplinary approach to treatment. Because of the complex, demanding, and long-term nature of recovery, it would be important to find a physician to manage the entire process. The strategy made sense but was frustrating, as I never could find a doctor to fill that role in the months of my recovery process.

My podiatrist, who had diagnosed the condition, specialized in surgery. He freely acknowledged that he had a tendency not to look beyond the foot in the healing process. It was hard to discuss anything beyond X rays and medications, much less the need for psychological support, spiritual resources, and the details of physical therapy exercises. My family doctor was empathetic to the challenges of chronic pain and was familiar with some of the medications used with CRPS but didn't seem to have an interest in overseeing treatment. Her practice was busy. The HMO doctors I visited were bound by company policies to limit time spent with patients, and some refused to keep current on the literature about CRPS. The time needed to develop and discuss the myriad strategies for healing was not part of the HMO plan. I consulted once with a knowledgeable physician at the University of Washington Pain Center, but he was not taking on new patients and the commute to Seattle meant taking too much time off work for each visit. The physical therapy professor who worked with me was the closest I had to a manager. He stayed with me until I was able to accomplish all functional goals for living sixteen months after developing CRPS, and he gave helpful feedback about the medications and nerve blocks I considered during the months of treatment. My pastor was familiar with some of my medical options because of chronic pain experiences he shared. He was the only professional with whom I could discuss my theological issues and spiritual disciplines used in recovery.

In the end, I managed my own recovery. I followed quota-based physical therapy exercise under the guidance of a competent therapist, elevated and massaged my foot two to three times a day, meditated twice a day, began a chronic pain support group that integrated spiritual practices into the healing process, taught a class for my congregation about suffering and faith, read books about others who were able to transform difficult life challenges into something valuable, spoke with others who had overcome the symptoms of CRPS, made a covenant for prayer and conversation with my pastor, and enjoyed the humor and compassion of family and friends.

It was lonely not having one person who understood it all. Even if I had found someone to manage it, he or she may not have truly understood the feelings I brought to the experience. However, managing on my own recovery, in hindsight, was a blessing. It meant I took charge of my own healing. Managing on my own never meant being alone. I found a whole community of support. I got to know many who taught me the art of healing in their own way as I moved from fear to hope, and from relentless pain to an active life again.

So you have found your doctor and, finally, a diagnosis. While identifying these two things would never seem a triumph in everyday life, it solves the first two pieces of the CRPS puzzle, and this usually happens after an often frantic and prolonged search. To many CRPS patients, it can present an oddly welcome moment of relief. Then the work begins.

Here's the next step: Create a plan of action, *immediately*. In the next chapter, we will begin with treatment options your doctor and other specialists can provide to target CRPS.

Treatment
Options for CRPS

Since so many bodily systems and processes are involved in CRPS/RSD, many treatment angles exist for tackling the condition. Moreover, what works for one patient might not have any effect for the next, so keeping an open mind about your options can help you and your doctor find the best combination. Experts now agree that multidisciplinary treatment—incorporating various elements of physical and psychological wellness efforts—offers the best approach to taking control of CRPS.

Treatment needs to come as early as possible, as the most successful means of arresting CRPS is identifying and controlling it in its early stages. Prompt, simultaneous, integrated treatment can intervene early enough to prevent temporary dysfunction from becoming permanent. Finally, CRPS symptoms can change for better or worse in a highly volatile fashion, so monitoring treatment effectively requires very careful, time-intensive, almost daily assessment of the patient's condition. This chapter offers an overview of treatments currently used for CRPS.

Complementary Therapies

Complementary therapies have carried me through my CRPS experience and continue to sustain me as regular sources of support in my life. Modalities such as acupuncture (on unaffected places), counseling, massage, relaxation techniques, art therapy, and yoga holistically attune to your most sensitive needs and prop you up to weather the physical, mental, and emotional demands that CRPS makes of you. Moreover, as there is much still unknown about CRPS in the medical field, complementary therapies enable you to boost your own body's healing abilities while following one of the many conventional medical treatments at the same time.

Imagine you have fallen off a bicycle and lost your ability to balance and ride it again. CRPS has thrown you off that bike. Complementary therapy provides you with training wheels so you can remount and ride your bike until your body is able to balance on its own again. There is so much to say about this aspect of CRPS care that, rather than try to cover the topic here, I have devoted an entire chapter to it. Chapter 6 describes the complementary approaches available to treat CRPS.

Physical and Occupational Therapy

Getting your affected areas moving again is critical in regaining and maintaining normal function. Physical therapy can help you improve range of motion of joints, improve motor control, and introduce normal functioning. Forget what you know about traditional repetitive-exercise sports physical therapy; as CRPS therapy includes practices for desensitizing your skin, manual therapy (massage) to relieve muscle spasms and edema, and education on regaining and adapting your activities of daily living. You can also request that the physical therapist show you exercises and desensitization practices for you to continue on your own at home.

Therapy can take place in a traditional office setting or in a pool of lukewarm water (82° to 93°F/28° to 34°C), which adds the extra benefit of soothing warmth that can relax muscles, support them, and alleviate the pressure of bearing weight on lower limbs. It is often said that things hurt less when done in warm water.

However, if you're sensitive even to the pressure of water, consider this an option you can revisit at a later time. Consider your relationship with water to be an ongoing, changing process in terms of tolerance of temperature and activity; it is a fine line to repeatedly tweak. For example, I personally could not tolerate the pressure of placing my hands underwater; this is one of the ways that I originally knew something was very wrong with my body. After a half year of CRPS treatments, I returned to the pool to tolerate fifteen to twenty minutes of gentle therapeutic movement before finger puckering would cause nerve sensitivity beyond my comfort zone. Having once taught swimming and been a summer lifeguard as a teen, I found myself using flotation aids to compensate for strength, trying the pool repeatedly while pushing away pride and grief. Seven years after my diagnosis, I returned to swimming regular laps. From this, I learned never to give up on something that may be temporary. Simply track your progress, be open to what works that day, and aim to eventually move into doing some regular swimming.

Crucially, physical therapy presents a very thin line for patients to walk between the pain from excessive activity and the pain from excessive inactivity. How can inactivity cause pain? Extended rest activates what are called *sleeping nociceptors,* which are deep-seated nerve endings that originate severe pain messages. At no time should you be pushed to achieve an external goal that causes excess stress to your body; rather, it is best to alternate between frequent movement and rest and slowly increase your tolerance levels for flexibility, motor control, and aerobic activity. Depending on any underlying injuries, such as a nerve entrapment or sprained ankle, your physical therapy may vary in rigorousness to prevent exacerbation of the problem. Keep in mind this is a long, slow path that requires patience and a learning curve for achieving balanced improvement. Finding an informed therapist who works in close coordination with your doctor and supports you in achieving this therapeutic middle ground is important for success.

Occupational therapy can help show you new ways to function at home, school, or work amid physical challenges and protect you against further injury while doing so. Your occupational therapist may brainstorm adaptive equipment to aid you in some functional tasks. For information on finding a physical therapist, see the Resources section. For more information on occupational therapy, read Chapter 6, "A World of Support: Complementary Therapies."

Mary's story demonstrates the importance of physical therapy as part of a complete treatment program for RSD/CRPS.

Mary's Story

In April 1999 I was riding my horse on a trail ride. When we stopped for a break, I decided to tie my horse to a fence post so I could go for a soda. The horse was jumpy, and I was distracted. As I was making the knot on the fence post, the horse spooked and reared back. My hand was caught in the knot between the horse and the fence post, which had been pulled out of the ground. Fearing the worst, I gritted my teeth and pulled my hand free, leaving parts of my ring and index finger behind and my thumb a mangled mess. I was rushed to the hospital, where I sat for four hours waiting for a hand specialist. By the time the doctor arrived, the situation was grim; he was unsure if he could reattach my thumb because of the nature of the injury and the time that had elapsed since the accident, but recommended attempting surgery. I had two failed surgeries (eight-plus hours each) in two days, after which I lost my thumb also.

About five weeks into my recovery, I started physical therapy (a.k.a. "physical torture"). My hand had been almost totally immobile during the preceding weeks. The physical therapy was extremely painful. No one could figure out why my little finger, which was not injured, was painful and difficult to move. When my hand started swelling after therapy, ice was recommended—but it made the pain much worse. My fingers looked like red, fat sausages, and my wrist started to stiffen. The physical therapy was so painful that I quit for a week, pending my next doctor's appointment.

When I returned to the hand specialist, he immediately recognized the problem as RSD/CRPS and made a referral to an anesthesiologist. The hand specialist didn't give me much information on the condition but did emphasize that I needed immediate treatment and ongoing PT. Once home, I started looking up RSD on the Internet and was devastated by what I found. The situation seemed hopeless. A few days later, I went to the anesthesiologist. He recommended a tricyclic antidepressant, as well as Neurontin and codeine-based medications. I was scheduled for a series of stellate ganglion blocks [upper-extremity sympathetic nerve blocks; see below] the next week. The meds had an immediate effect; I was able to sleep for the first time in months.

After the first block, I immediately resumed PT. It was slow and painful, but tolerable, as I finally had a physical therapist who understood RSD. The therapist prepared me for therapy by starting with a wax bath to heat up the hand and wrist—then proceeded to work with passive motion until I was able to move on my own. She also used some type of sonogram therapy and a TENS unit. [For more about TENS units, see Chapter 6.] I was later referred to a physical medicine specialist for additional therapy and pain management. I slowly started to get better.

When I returned to the anesthesiologist, he seemed disappointed with my progress and suggested that surgery to sever the nerves might be needed. I asked for a second opinion, and he refused to continue my treatment, stating that if I did not have confidence in his recommendations, he could not continue to be my doctor. I was shocked. I returned to the physical medicine specialist and requested that he take over my case. He agreed. We continued with PT, and he referred me for biofeedback training. The biofeedback helped me with pain control, and I was able to start tapering off of the pain meds. My hand and wrist were now working, but my shoulder had become partially immobile (hand/shoulder syndrome). I started PT for the shoulder. I thought it would never end.

Fifteen months after my accident, I went into full remission. I have complete use of what is left of my hand, and I am pain-free.

Since then, I have broken my leg, my collarbone, and a rib (horsing around)—but have experienced no relapse.

I credit my recovery to the quick diagnosis by my hand specialist, an accurate and experienced anesthesiologist, an understanding physical therapist, and a physical medicine specialist who listened.

Mirror Box Therapy

Mirror therapy can be practiced with your doctor or physical therapist and has been shown to help activate the frontal cortex to rewire the brain, particularly in the acute stages of CRPS. By positioning a mirror perpendicular to you and only exposing your unaffected extremity in the reflection, moving that limb can help to support rewiring of your nervous system as the painless limb moves and appears in the place of the painful one. Pre-imagining movement exercises may support this practice, before the mirror is used. This practice is used not only on CRPS patients but also on military amputees experiencing phantom-limb pain.

Drug Therapy

Because many different neurotransmitters (e.g. substance P, serotonin, prostaglandins, bradykinin, leukotrienes, histamine) and receptors (e.g., opioid, serotonin, acetylcholine, dopamine, norepinephrine) are involved in pain, several drug therapies are used to treat CRPS. While drug therapy does not cure RSD, it can optimize pain control and provide the relief necessary to regain function and participate in other therapies. Many drugs used in treating CRPS are currently prescribed for "off-label" use. In other words, they may be approved by the U.S. Food and Drug Administration to treat one condition, but doctors also use the drug to treat another condition, such as CRPS. Each drug category is reviewed below.

Anticonvulsants

Anticonvulsants such as Neurontin (gabapentin), Tegretol (carbamazepine), Lyrica (pregabalin), and Dilantin (phenytoin) work by stabilizing the nerve membranes and controlling random neuron "firing." They can ease the sensations of burning, electric shocks, stabbing, or jerking nerve pain. Gabapentin offers fewer side effects than other options and interacts well with many medications; it depresses excitatory mechanisms and has also showed in studies to support the effects of other pain-relieving adjuvant therapies. However, since each medication controls neuron firing via different routes, a multi-medication approach is often recommended to halt the progression of CRPS from peripheral nerve routes to the central nervous system.

Tricyclic Antidepressants

Tricyclic antidepressants such as Pamelor (nortriptyline) and Elavil (amitriptyline) increase the uptake of certain neurotransmitters that provide pain relief and improve sleep. Amitriptyline has been the most widely used analgesic until now; however, it can be very sedating to patients, cause hypotension, and spark significant weight gain—a side effect particularly risky when patients are already struggling to bear weight on their feet.

Transdermal Medications

Anesthetic and opioid medications such as Lidoderm (lidocaine) and Duragesic (fentanyl) can be absorbed by the skin via a patch, avoiding complications associated with their oral administration and systemic absorption. More controversially, patients can seek topical pain relief and gradual desensitization with capsaicin, the natural substance that makes chili peppers so hot. While initially causing increased pain that may be unbearable in the case of CRPS, continued use of capsaicin cream reduces the amount of substance P, which plays a role in transmission of pain messages. Convenient for symptomatic relief, these medications can be applied according to pain needs. Clonidine patches and ketamine cream are also options. For more information on ketamine, see NMDA-receptor antagonists.

Mary Ann's story discusses her use of the prescription cream Ketocaine 60 with PLO 20, in combination with physical therapy.

ary Ann's Story

I was diagnosed with CRPS/RSD in February 2003. I had broken my right wrist and was in a cast from November 29 til January 18. When the cast came off, all I had was an appendage that would not move, looked like five sausages, and was red. I was started on physical therapy three times a week when my hand was still swollen. It was extremely painful. I could barely get my thumb to touch the side of my index finger, much less the tip of it.

My physical therapist was the one who noticed the shininess of my skin and the black hairs that had started to show up on my right hand. He advised me to look up RSD on the computer and he [did] some research as well. Though my orthopedic physician had told me I had to do the physical therapy strenuously every day or I would lose the use of my hand, my physical therapist and I worked out an alternative routine that was not too strenuous (which would just exacerbate the symptoms). It was methodical in the stretching exercises for the tendons, which were done each day at home in addition to at the two sessions I had each week at the physical therapist's office. I cried a lot doing the exercises, but I did them because I was afraid I'd lose the use of the hand forever. It did not even feel like a hand.

A friend told me about a compounded medicine he had been prescribed for his shoulder: Ketocaine 60 with PLO 20. I told my MD about it, and he prescribed it for me. Just a little bit of the cream rubbed on each of the joints in my fingers and my wrist, and ten minutes later I could move them better and farther without pain! This was a miracle drug to me. The more my hand and fingers were able to move, the less shiny the hand became. I also experienced a reduction of the episodes of pain radiating from my fingertips to my elbow.

I went through eighteen treatments of physical therapy, then an additional eighteen. My hand is now functional. I am typing, crocheting, rolling my own hair, etc. My hand and wrist are not perfect. I cannot make a fist, but I can hold a potato peeler. I cannot push myself up from the bathtub with my right hand but I can lift the corner of the mattress and tuck in sheets. I have done strength training with a squeeze ball and then a grip device to which you add rubber bands to tighten the resistance. I did sensitivity training so that I could stand the feel of jeans or even a dishcloth in my right hand.

I don't know what winter will bring. I used to have to wear a glove in temperatures below 62°F or so. My right hand would feel like it was in a freezer and hurt. I have now developed an allergy to the Ketocaine that causes little blisters on my skin, but I know that I wouldn't have gotten back this much use of my hand without it. I have to do stretching exercises every day to keep the hand mobile, so I run warm water over my hands to loosen them up or use my hot wax bath on them. I feel that I am licking the disease or at least keeping it from being debilitating. I have come off the Tylox and am taking Advil only for pain.

Take note here that Mary Ann's topical medication was a compounded prescription. In other words, the drug was not specifically approved and available for use in the United States, but this formula was specifically mixed by a compounding pharmacy with a prescription from her doctor. Compounding pharmacies legally create custom-made medications for patients when mass-produced and approved drug alternatives are not deemed appropriate or effective. Compounded medications can carry with them additional risks because they have not been evaluated in clinical trials (by the country in which you live) for their particular dosage and combination. Yet, your doctor may find that such tailor-made medications are worth the risk for serving your particular treatment needs. You can find more information on pharmacy compounding in the Resources section.

Calcium Channel Blockers

Medications such as nifedipine and amlodipine enable increased blood flow to the heart and relax the blood vessels so that blood flows more easily to the extremities where circulation may be challenged.

NMDA Receptor Antagonists

Glutamate is a neurotransmitter in the central nervous system and spinal cord that is thought to play a role in the transmission and perception of pain. Under certain conditions of intense or prolonged pain, such as those that can occur after a physical injury, glutamate released from sensory nerves appears to be able to create "windup" and central nervous system sensitization; in other words, the central nervous system overreacts to normal sensory input or may even spontaneously generate sensations (oftentimes painful) that do not even exist. It appears to do this, at least in part, by excessively stimulating postsynaptic sites in the spinal cord and thalamus that are referred to as N-methyl-D-aspartate (NMDA) receptors. In such a case, the stimulation spontaneously stays active long after the fading away of glutamate that was released by the injury. Why does this happen? Under certain conditions, once the NMDA receptors are switched on by the glutamate, the receptors act as if they have become "jammed" in the "on" position, and there is nothing in the body that seems to be strong enough to turn them "off."

Ketamine, an anesthetic approved by the Food and Drug Administration (FDA), is an NMDA-receptor antagonist, which means that it appears to be able to block some of the effects of glutamate and turn "off" the NMDA receptors. Originally developed in the 1960s to be used as an intravenous anesthetic, it was found to have very analgesic effects—but came with hallucinogenic and psychological side effects. In the decades that followed ketamine's waning use as an intravenous anesthetic, many researchers and physicians began to find other uses for ketamine—especially as a drug to treat pain. It can be administered in conjunction with other drugs to decrease the likelihood or intensity of its side effects.

Ketamine infusion treatments conducted in Germany and Mexico have featured "deep ketamine anesthesia," in which a continuous intravenous infusion of ketamine and another drug, such as midazolam, induces a deep sedation state in patients for more than five days. Side effects such as hallucinations, increased heart rate, anxiety, increased blood pressure, and delirium have occurred in some patients, and serious safety issues can arise as part of the treatment. For this extreme approach, severe, advanced CRPS patients decide that the benefits outweigh the risks in pursuing this path; overall, many patients have responded with reduction in pain and, particularly, diminution of allodynia by essentially "resetting" the nervous system while in a medical coma. Longer-term tracking has indicated that booster infusion sessions (while awake) have been required to manage relapse and recurrent or residual pain.

Meanwhile, Dr. Ronald Harbut, in collaboration with Dr. Graeme Correll of Australia, pioneered the sub-anesthetic low-dose ketamine treatment, or "awake technique," during which a patient remains awake while receiving intravenous ketamine. This method involves much lower doses than with the coma approach and has demonstrated meaningful relief in about 30 to 50 percent of patients. Follow-up infusions may be part of a patient's longer-term management of CRPS to maintain the effects, which have included both pain reduction and functional improvement. Ketamine has also been shown to support and maintain positive vasodilative effects when coupled with a stellate ganglion blockade.

Since the original publication of this book, ketamine treatment has become more widespread, for both patients with pain unresponsive to other treatments and for those who seek alternatives. Topical creams, oral pills, sublingual lozenges, and a nasal spray containing ketamine have also been cited by doctors and patients as helpful to reducing neuropathic pain. It must be handled and stored carefully, as it is a controlled substance and an abused street drug. U.S. military medical professionals have used ketamine infusions to treat some soldiers suffering severe pain from massive blast injuries. The low-dose ketamine technique or coma inducement offer possible treatment alternatives for appropriate patients when conventional treatments are unsuccessful, contraindicated, or not well tolerated by the patient. Hopefully, this treatment option will receive the relevant insurance coverage it deserves. Below is a story from Barby, who found significant relief with ketamine subanesthetic intravenous infusions:

Barby's Story

I have been battling CRPS since September 2002. I know firsthand how hard it is to continue looking for relief and answers, and coming up against health-care professionals who blow you off—or do not believe what you are describing could actually be what you are experiencing. After seeing over one hundred health-care professionals, getting major surgeries I did not need, having complications such as internal bleeding, medication interactions, kidney stones, tumors growing in my mouth, and so much more, I did not give up or give in!

In December 2009 I achieved remission after undergoing inpatient IV-ketamine infusions and follow-up boosters. I literally went into the hospital in a wheelchair and walked out seven days later. I undergo two-day booster infusions approximately every four months.

My infusion cocktail includes clonidine, Ativan, versed, and Zofran, so I don't have hallucinations, and I also don't remember anything for two days after a booster. So a booster lasts four days for me. I have hope that more doctors will begin to do the ketamine infusion protocol that helped me go from wheels to heels.

A lot of people think remission means: "Done; I get my life back now." Most people do not realize that remission is a new experience all in itself. Going into Drexel for my infusions, I felt, "Here is my time, my chance, my everything, to possibly reverse what I have been living with since 2002." I believed deep down that ketamine infusions would put me into remission. My excitement was great, along with the rest of my family's. My regular treating doctors were not so optimistic, but not discouraging either.

Once I arrived back home, I went to visit my primary care physician. He was shocked at how I was doing. He did not think it was going to work. I had a glow of life that he had NEVER seen since he first began treating me in May 2005. He opened the exam room door and called the nurses and office staff. "Come look at Barby. I can't believe how she is doing," he said. They came in and were shocked as well. He and his staff never knew me before reflex sympathetic dystrophy. They were now looking at the "after ketamine Barby" and were so happy for me.

I am a new person. I'm not the same person I was eleven years ago, but who is the same person they were eleven years ago? Whether physical or mental, pain can and will consume you, if you allow it to. Whether you have been in remission or are still dreaming of it, know that it will be a new chapter in life, and expecting the same life you always knew before your CRPS set in may not be so realistic. Remission is fulfilling, hopeful, and a great experience, but it was not exactly as I expected. I've learned that chronic conditions such as complex regional pain syndrome are lifelong changers.

Opiates

Opiate agonists such as morphine, codeine, Percocet, and Darvon are used for relieving the most severe pain by imitating and enhancing the naturally occurring chemicals in the central nervous system that inhibit pain messages among neurons. Agonists also act as sedatives, reducing central nervous system activity and enabling sleep, but they also can cause excessive drowsiness. Users can run the risk of becoming dependent or of developing a tolerance to therapeutic levels. They also potentially interfere with immune functions, as well as memory and physical function. However, since some patients obtain significant pain relief with opioids (and therefore significantly increased function, which is the primary goal of treatment), testing and using them should *not* be delayed as a "last resort." Oftentimes the efforts made to prevent the abuse and street sale of prescription drugs in the United States has unfortunately infringed upon sufficient prescription of opioids for CRPS patients.

An alternative to opioid agonists is buprenorphine, an opioid agonist-antagonist that provides analgesic ease without the risks of dependency or depression. Many trials testing opiates are ongoing. For more information, you can flip to the Resources section of this book.

Bisphosphonates

Neridronate is a very promising drug with results just recently published from its multi-center, randomized, double-blind placebo-controlled trial. Of eighty-two patients with acute CRPS-1 in an extremity treated with four IV infusions of the drug, the results were significant and long lasting. Due to the success of the treatment, even placebo participants were then given the opportunity to receive neridronate treatment. Resolution of CRPS symptoms was confirmed with all participants a year later. At the time of this book edition, the drug is under U.S. FDA review to be approved specifically for CRPS. Let's hope it will be on the market and covered by insurance by the time you read this.

Anti-Inflammatories

NSAIDs, or nonsteroidal anti-inflammatory drugs, can help treat the swelling and inflammation involved in many CRPS cases, though they carry the risk of gastric bleeding if used for an extended time. They come in prescription form, as well as over-the-counter medication such as ibuprofen.

Antispasmodics

Medications such as baclofen and clonazepam can be used to ease muscle spasms and contractures, via an oral dosage or more potent delivery via intrathecal pump.

Free-Radical Scavengers

It is thought that free radicals play a role in the excessive inflammatory response to trauma and immune system impairment that is seen in CRPS. Dimethylsulfoxide (DMSO) is a standard treatment for early CRPS patients (less than one year) in the Netherlands. In some studies it has been shown to help treat redness, swelling, and pain when applied topically. N-acetyl-cysteine (NAC) has also offered good results for patients suffering "cold" and CRPS symptoms; DMSO is more effective on "warm" CRPS symptoms. Vitamin C has shown to help reduce the development of CRPS in wrist fracture patients.

Corticosteroids

Administered in oral form before contractures appear in a CRPS patient, initial treatment of swelling and an excessively warm limb with methylprednisone—which is quickly tapered—offers a possible alternative to a more invasive nerve-block procedure. The risks of corticosteroid use, such as gastrointestinal ulcers, weight gain, and heightened blood pressure should also be thoroughly considered with corticosteroid use.

Other Promising Drugs Reportedly Tested

Intravenous immunoglobulin (IVIG) was shown to benefit a small number of CPRS patients in a study, confirming the immune system involvement in the condition. IVIG has shown similar efficacy to other lower-cost options, including ketamine.

Intravenous blocks using TNF-x antibodies were reported to have positive results, revealing the need for controlled studies.

Nerve Blocks

There are three types of nerve blockades, all of which use anesthetics such as lidocaine or bretylium to achieve their pain-relieving effects. Relieving pain can help patients get into a physical therapy routine, tolerate touch, and simultaneously calm down the neurons affected.

Regional Sympathetic Blocks

These anesthetics are commonly administered to treat early CRPS, as pain is still considered to be significantly under the control of the sympathetic nervous system at this stage. They also help increase temperature in a cold extremity. In addition, they can help determine how much pain is associated with the sympathetic nervous system, which enables your doctor to decide on a treatment plan for you, depending on the response. The blocks are usually administered as a series of three injections and consist of the injection of local anesthetic into the back of the neck or lower back, depending on whether the upper or lower extremities are affected. Prolonged sympathetic blocks have also had excellent results for patients at times. In more-advanced stages of CRPS, regional sympathetic blocks can lose their effectiveness, with continued debate surrounding how many blocks are too many.

Responsiveness to sympathetic blocks has often been used to confirm the diagnosis of CRPS. However, just because a patient does not respond to a sympathetic block *does not mean that she or he does not have CRPS*. Pain, especially in patients who have had symptoms for a significant period of time, can become independent of the sympathetic nervous system, and CRPS is also a central nervous system disease.

Intravenous Regional Blocks

Anesthesia medications can also be administered by IV into the affected area to numb the pain locally. Different medications can be used to target either the sympathetic nervous system or somatic nervous systems.

Epidural Blocks

Just as epidural anesthesia is administered to ease the pain of childbirth, it can also be used to block pain via insertion of a small catheter into the spinal canal. Anesthesia is then injected through this route to reach pain receptors in the spinal cord.

Stefanie, a brave young person whose story follows, experienced great success with nerve block treatment, among other therapies, such as desensitization. While not every CRPS patient has the level of success with nerve blocks that Stefanie enjoyed, her story is a good example of how effective the treatment can be in some cases.

S *tefanie's Story*

My name is Stefanie, and I am twelve years old. I developed RSD in my left foot in January 2003. I think it was a sprain because I did not break anything. At first, my foot hurt really badly, and so I iced and elevated it, thinking that the pain would go away in a day or two. But it just got worse. At the time, I had been playing soccer and basketball and was in my fourth year dancing jazz and hip-hop.

As the pain got worse, my mom took me to the doctor to get an X ray. It showed inflammation but nothing else. By this time the skin on my foot had started to peel, and my foot was turning blue and cold. I had two MRIs, and once again they showed nothing. The pain was so bad that I couldn't even walk on my foot! Putting on my shoe was so hard because my foot was so sensitive to touch.

The doctor said that my foot was hurt from overuse and told me to stay off it. When that didn't work, a cast was put on it. That was when my mom took me for a second opinion. This doctor took off the cast and right away knew what I had. It was called reflex sympathetic dystrophy or complex regional pain syndrome. He told me that he could help me and that the pain I was having was extremely bad and he knew how hard it was to put my foot down. However, the nerve messages from my brain were sending faulty messages to my foot, saying that there was something wrong with the foot when in reality there was not. The doctor said if there was any way I could start using my foot, I would get better faster.

I still could not put my foot on the floor; the doctor couldn't even touch my foot because it hurt so much. So he ordered physical therapy and prescribed Neurontin 100 mg and Advil. My foot was swollen, blue, cold, and sensitive to touch, and I was on crutches, not walking on it at all.

My mom borrowed a foot massager from a neighbor and started putting my foot in it. At first, the water made my foot hurt so badly. "But you know everything hurts your foot. Just try to keep it in the water," she said. I put my headphones on and blasted my music, and then I managed to keep my foot in the massager for five minutes. Later on, I was able to keep it in for ten and then twenty minutes, until I could keep it in for hours. The massager made my foot feel better and did not hurt it. The color of my foot would turn to pink instead of blue and the temperature of my foot would become warm again. So I continued this every day, sometimes three times a day. Whenever my mom saw my foot blue or cold, she would get the massager. Finally, I could tolerate bubbles and jets, and the massager was helping the sensitivity in my foot. After the massager, I would rub and dry my foot with a towel; it would hurt, but I still did it to try to desensitize it.

I started going to physical therapy, putting my foot in a Jacuzzi and then doing exercises to strengthen my foot and leg because I had lost a lot of muscle. By May, I started seeing some results. I was riding an exercise bike, doing more strengthening exercises, and starting to get my balance back little by little. It was so hard to do all the things that I had to do, but I did all of it. Sometimes I just wanted to cry, but I knew that I had to do it to get better. My mom was always there, cheering me on, or holding my hand. Soon, I was on one crutch—and then no crutches!

By August of 2003 my left leg had as much muscle as my right leg did, and my foot no longer turned colors or got cold. I could walk on my foot, but I had trouble running. I continued PT three times a week, but I did not play soccer, basketball, or dance; instead, I rode horseback and was pretty good at it. I also rode my bike, played tag, and was in less pain than I used to be.

I went to see a new doctor—a pain-management doctor—in September, and we decided he would do a regional nerve block. I had one nerve block and when I awoke, I felt no pain. My back was a little sore, but it was nothing compared to the pain I had with RSD. I rested for a few hours and then was up, walking around, with no pain. A few hours later, I was so excited because the nerve block worked. After a week, I started getting flashes of pain in my foot. They would come and go, but they were very painful. I told my mom, and she made an appointment for a second nerve block. I had the second nerve block a week later. The nerve block worked again, and I have been pain-free since then.

I am still pain-free. I would definitely recommend nerve blocks as a way to get rid of the pain. I know for some it does not work, but for me, it has given me my life back. I feel like the luckiest girl in the world. I am horseback riding and playing gym in school with no limitations once again. I am so excited to finally be able to run, laugh, and play again.

For all of you who are reading this and know of someone who has RSD/CRPS, or if you have it yourself, try really hard to work through the pain and never feel like the pain is in your head or that you're crazy. *The pain is real.* If you know of someone who has RSD, just remain the same friend you were before RSD. You may have to do different things, like go to the movies or watch TV instead of running and playing sports, but be there for that person.

Surgical Treatments

Surgical procedures should never be rushed into, but it is good to know what some doctors are considering using further down the road. Weigh any surgical steps carefully with your doctor, and ask for his or her success rates, along with risk estimates with your particular type of CRPS.

Sympathectomy

This is now considered a controversial approach to blocking pain, and it includes extremely high risks for additional tissue damage and spread of CRPS. With the aim of obstructing pain, chemical, radiofrequency and surgical sympathectomies essentially "kill" or mechanically cut the sympathetic nerves responsible for the affected area.

As CRPS can be exacerbated and spread by invasive treatments and nerve damage, the risks found to be associated with these approaches must be thoroughly examined, and you should always seek a second or third opinion. While some practitioners still advocate partial sympathectomy for the lower extremities, others have stopped performing them. Some discourage radiofrequency and chemical sympathectomies but advocate surgical sympathectomy; others, such as Dr. Hooshmand Hooshang, have literally advised that "a sympathectomy, be it surgical or chemical, is useless for your advanced RSD. It will cause rapid spread of your CRPS to other parts of the body." Sympathectomy also potentially precludes future new treatments from working.

Undoubtedly, the patient who can benefit from this treatment must be carefully selected, and any patient considering it needs to be aware of the procedure's risks. Further, only those who have been receptive to sympathetic blocks should be considered.

Implantable Devices

These devices dispense medication or stimulation continually to provide pain relief in the most serious of intractable pain cases. With implanted drip-irrigation medication pumps, intraspinal drug infusions block pain signals to the brain by using narcotics, such as morphine or dilaudid, to reach certain receptors in the spinal cord. With a pump, a much smaller dose is needed to reach the spinal fluid than would be necessary orally, thereby decreasing side effects. Baclofen pumps have proven effective in blocking movement disorder.

Spinal cord stimulators (SCS) use low intensity, electrical impulses to interrupt and even stop pain signals from being transferred to the brain. The result is a constant tingling sensation, called *paresthesia*, along the spinal cord and throughout the body. A trial procedure with a temporary electrode can be done to evaluate the effectiveness before the actual stimulator is surgically implanted. A follow-up study evaluating SCS patients over the course of two years has been positive, both for significant pain reduction and improved overall quality of life for both cervical and lumbar SCS implantation. Anecdotal evidence has suggested that stimulators can sometimes eventually calm down hyperexcitable neurons along the spinal cord. It's important to note that this is still an invasive, risky procedure.

If the above treatments fail to prove effective, do not consider this the end of your options, as both new and experimental treatments are becoming available for CRPS sufferers. Some drugs listed in this chapter, for example, may not yet be offered to patients on a widespread basis. However, in the open call for more-effective therapies, treatment alternatives are available to you if you're willing to track down a doctor administering them. In addition, Chapter 6 of this book will introduce you to complementary therapies, which can greatly support you and help reduce your pain *in tandem with* conventional medicine. Finally, you can find information on clinical trials in the Resources section.

Scrambler Therapy

This newer computer-generated electrotherapy option operates on the premise of delivering transdermal "nonpain" information to patients' painful areas to block their pain signals. Delivering a sequence of various nerve action potentials that simulate endogenous ones, the Scrambler technology relies on electrodes to send these pain-modulating pulses via noninvasive skin patches. Scrambler therapy was developed in Italy and differs from transcutaneous electrical nerve stimulation, or TENS (see Chapter 6) by providing nonlinear, continuously variable information, while TENS delivers consistent, linear electrical information to a patient's subcutaneous nerves. Branded as the Calmare Pain Therapy Medical Device, it is FDA 510(k)–cleared for severe neuropathic pain treatment and has shown positive and lasting results in CRPS and neuropathic pain patients.

Prognosis

Is there a "cure" for CRPS? No. Not yet! Can people recover or go into remission? Yes. With early treatment, ideally within the first three months of onset, CRPS can potentially be arrested within the first stage or improved, while more advanced stages of the disease might be pushed back to a milder form. CRPS tends to be an unpredictable disease, which makes its outcome possess both frightening uncertainties as well as triumphant possibilities for recovery. Much has happened in the past decade of research. Perhaps the ultimate future may rest in genetic therapies that could induce the return of the hypersensitized spinal cord to normal.

Realizing that so much is unknown about CRPS, one must also consider the possibility for progress, and that hope and opportunity for improvement is the focus of this book. In the meantime, while you guard your faith in the future, you can do many things *right now* to enable the greatest ease and quality of life possible with CRPS. From this launching pad, let's jump into the next chapter and get started.

Tips for Body and Soul

Living with CRPS will lead you to new discoveries about your problem-solving skills, community resources, and personal inventiveness. Sometimes a simple movement or activity, such as putting away laundry or opening a bag of frozen food, will seem insignificant as a single, isolated action; however, the sum of every little action or movement of the day can leave you overexerted and exhausted. The key to handling your new body is to support it during both painful *and* regular activity. Because CRPS is now believed to affect the entire body, you must seize every opportunity to support your new body's heightened needs, giving it more chances to heal and replenish itself for challenges that are presently too painful to pursue. Ultimately, you will safeguard your function in current activities and increase the chances of resuming those activities that you have cut out completely.

Equally important are ways to distract your mind, find a place for it to play, and temporarily escape the pressures placed on your patience and well-being by your symptoms. Starting over or mentally escaping can breathe new energy and fortitude into your spirit, acting as a buffer against CRPS anxiety. Is this escapism? Let's remove the stigma from that word when addressing intense chronic pain and call it an opportunity for mental expansion that is medically beneficial. Amid your physical limitations, explore the boundaries of your consciousness and *use whatever works for you.* There are no wrong methods or ways on this path, so channel your desperation or shock into creating a game, a mantra, a visual memory, or a meditation that speaks to your soul. Use it to stretch your "inner place" of safety, to cradle and nurture your suffering spirit.

Below, you will find plenty of ways to make your life easier, as well as many ways to feel inspired if you're "stuck" and looking for a pick-me-up or stress releaser. Flip through the list of suggestions below and try them on for size.

Activity Modifications

You can make many functional modifications to reduce the stress on your body during daily activity, and each adaptation will save a bit more energy for you to handle your CRPS symptoms. Whether it be a behavioral change or a new technology, each of these elements below is a step you can take right now to feel more control over your quality of life.

Guard Your Central Nervous System

Since your nervous system and excitotoxicity (neuron-damaging overactivity in the form of spasms or attacks) are involved in CRPS, finding ways to keep calm can support your physical well-being. Consider that your arousal level can affect the volume level of your pain. You may have been a fearless socialite or horror-movie fan before CRPS, but now you need to regard yourself as a person in shock who must gently reintroduce yourself to stimuli in the world around you. Avoiding large events, loud sounds, suspenseful or frightening movies, strong vibrations, and intense or panicky people can spare your system a lot of excess stimulation. Use this as a chance to understand a quieter, core you. Revamp your musical tastes and experiment with soft, calming, and smooth music rather than high-energy or jumpy tunes. As you get to know your body, you may dip your foot back into higher-intensity environments and gradually set new limits.

Keep a Pain Journal

"Keep a diary of all my pains? Don't I think about that enough all day?" Yes, the last thing you probably wish to do is focus on the subject that most troubles you, but keeping a detailed record of your symptoms and pain level can empower you to participate in your recuperation. Your journal history is your voice and the key to your personal recovery. Neither you—nor your doctor—will remember as much as you think you will concerning your medical history, and different medical treatments vary in effectiveness from person to person. Additionally, the diffuse nature of CRPS can cause your symptoms to shift, so a brief, constantly updated log can help you note pain patterns with regard to medication, healing therapies, rest, and specific activities over time.

Journaling your pain enables you to voice it succinctly, validate it, and put it away somewhere outside of your head—for the day. Moreover, recording your pain levels and completed activities provides a way for you to see the baby steps of improvement you make over time. Record your accomplishments, too! On a day when the same old burning and tingling keeps you from doing anything, remove yourself from self-destructive thoughts of exasperation and take a look at your diary to see how far you've come.

If you feel more comfortable organizing your CRPS history in a chart, here's a sample of my own original tracking. I included dates for every doctor and therapy appointment, as well as notable dates on which I was feeling better, had accomplished something new, experienced a setback, and so on. I often included specifics from therapy treatments to track their effect on how I feel. My most-used space was occupied by comments, rants, and joys. Finally, I included mileage or cost of transport to each medical appointment, along with the appointment date, which is helpful to track if you have workers' compensation.

Date	Event	Results	Comments	Cost of transport or mileage
8/12	Therapy with Sheri	Acupuncture on back. Massage on triceps; was told that trigger points in triceps are slowly coming out. Next time, work will begin on forearms and hands.	Still feel nerves and muscles are in spasm. Acupuncture released extra nervousness over chest and quieted body until midday. Accomplishments: took shower alone, sometimes dressing self, finally opening refrigerator with hands and not feet. Still need help with shoes, buttons, bras, preparing food, opening packages, using key to open doors. Can write little more beyond my signature. Some days can bend arms; other days elbows burn too much.	10.2 miles
10/1			Dressing self, opening some container lids, serving self from serving bowls, can write two to three lines by hand, lifted a light drink, and put on makeup! Evening: nerves feel stringy and hot all the way to elbow, strange shakiness, and loss of muscle control. Able to concentrate on books finally!	

Since I've gone into remission, my tracking format and details have changed. However, I relaunch them if I have a flare-up. I also have found that recording great strides and moments of feeling pain-free have helped me cope when I do revert back to chronic pain that I still manage daily; I read these over again to keep my "All is lost!" despair at bay.

Use Voice-Activated Software

If you have CRPS in your arms, voice-activated software may be your sole method of recording information, making lists, taking care of basic bureaucratic writing and organizational needs, and expressing yourself through journaling. If your problem is in your lower extremities, using the software can still be beneficial in re-serving your hands for other uses (e.g., wheelchair maneuvering) and saving them from the risk of computer-related repetitive stress injuries.

The latest version of Dragon NaturallySpeaking has made huge strides in accuracy, is simple to install, and can be purchased on-line for your convenience. Try www.Nuance.com, Amazon.com, or Bestbuy.com for a broad selection of voice-activated software and check into www.voicerecognition.net for pre-purchasing questions about your computer configuration. More experienced voice-activated software users can try eBay.com to snatch a deeply discounted upgrade.

You can even write a book with voice software these days. It's not easy, but it can be done: I wrote the original edition of this book with Dragon NaturallySpeaking Preferred, version 7. Voice software enabled me to return to a full-time office job, four years after I developed CRPS. It reduces my keyboarding needs by 60 percent and has been the essential key to rebuilding my career after I was well enough to work. I can also share with you the pit-falls and frustrations of trying to keep up on voice software—or to program and memorize necessary commands, as well. Yet one thing remains clear: This invention has bridged an enormous bar-rier. With smartphones now also using voice engines, these little wins are making life easier in significant ways I could only have dreamed of ten years ago.

Use a Headset

A headset can give your hands a bit of a rest or serve as the one and only lifeline to your friends and family if you're homebound. If your hands burn, yet you have to make phone calls to doctors, workers' compensation lawyers, and bill collectors, this minor tool can make the experience ten times less painful. If your fingers hurt, you can dial the phone with your big toe! Even now, holding the phone still hurts me after awhile. Every little bit helps.

Make Functional Aids a Mainstay

Functional tools made especially for people with medical challenges make it possible for you to take more control and be more independent around the house, even though you'll be doing things differently than you did before. For your benefit, online and mail-order catalogs make obtaining assistive devices as simple as purchasing them over the telephone. Catalogs offer a range of extremely helpful items, such as electric jar openers, cutting boards with prongs to hold food, claw-type pick-up sticks for reaching beyond your limits, pushable levers for turning keys and doorknobs, book holders with page turners, elastic shoelaces, walking sticks, electric knives, electric potato peelers, adaptive scissors, and so on. Moreover, if you're not completely wheelchair bound or cane dependent, using assistive devices at select times, even if it's only for specific events such as walking through a mall, should not be considered a "cop-out." Doing so helps you to save energy for the fun activities. Assistive devices do not have to become your identity.

To get started, check out the catalogs *Functional Solutions, Allegro Medical, Independent Living Aids, Inc.,* and others at the following websites:

www.infinitec.org/live/kitchens/catalogsaids.htm

www.ncmedical.com

www.hdis.com/mobility.html

More assistive-device resources are included in the Resources section in the back of the book.

Aim for Automatic

Find devices already available to the general public that will do things for you. Electric can openers, mini food processors, and electric staplers can greatly reduce strain on your hands. These days, a lightweight, portable, battery-powered toothbrush costs less than twenty dollars and saves your arms from repetitive, back-

and-forth motion. If your hands are sensitive to vibration, wrap the brush handle with a towel to lighten the sensation. Find one with an on/off switch to eliminate the need for you to continually press a button to keep it active.

Go Light

Switch to plastic cups, utensils, and plates to make lifting and handling items as easy as possible. You can also reduce the amount of washing required for dishes on a daily basis with disposable tableware. If it hurts too much to lift a cup, keep straws handy for hands-free drinking. Dishwasher-friendly and hot-liquid straws are mainstays at my home. Buy items such as detergent in smaller amounts, or have someone help you transfer products from heavy bulk containers into smaller dispensers.

Get It Delivered

While CRPS may be seriously draining your pockets, it can still be worth it to save your body a bit and get your groceries and other home supplies delivered. Often, if items are purchased in bulk, the cost of delivery can be roughly the same as going out and braving the store yourself. Check out Safeway, Peapod, or Publix online or see if your local grocer can arrange a delivery for you. As you heal and become more knowledgeable of adaptive aids and proper ways to support your body, you can venture out again for your own supplies.

Pamper Your Pain-Free Parts

Remember the other parts of your body that bring you pleasure and express your gratitude to them. Consider massage therapy to nourish these parts and remind your body of positive sensations, keeping your brain circuitry aware of normal nerve function. Massage can produce endorphins to help your body buffer pain, as well as increase circulation. Take your time and discover new areas that can please you: Get one foot, your scalp, or your lower back massaged.

Other physical touches that you might have dropped since CRPS arrived can also reinforce positive associations with your body. Spritz perfume on your unaffected skin and reinvite luxury into your self-perception. Get a manicure or pedicure, depending on which areas are healthy. Keep your skin well moisturized. CRPS is currently a part of you rather than a syndrome that affects just one region; cherishing and pampering your entire body can optimize healing.

Keep Warm

Always leave home well prepared with extra layers of clothing, and keep warm mittens and/or socks nearby. Your circulation can be challenged by CRPS itself and the inactivity it causes, and cold extremities can sharpen creepy-crawly, cold-knife pain in your extra-sensitive state.

Whenever you feel the sickliness of inactivity and cold, try to at least sway back-and-forth and move or stretch slowly to jump-start your circulation. Even if you move at a snail's pace, keep a "flow" going in your body to stay warm. Watch out for large meals, as the blood rush to the stomach, assisting in digestion, can even leave your hands and feet feeling extra sensitive.

Make Your Own Heating Pads

Think you need to pay a fortune for portable heating pads? Fill a thick, white sport sock with plain, white rice, and close the end tightly with a tie that does not include any metal or rubber. Pop it into the microwave for two minutes, and you have a homemade heating pad to warm sore, spasming muscles and rigid tendons. Even amid burning pain, the mild heat can often calm the frenetic activity in your hands and feet and provide relief for cold extremities—not to mention providing comfort that might restore and occupy your distressed self.

Test and Protect Your Sensitive Areas

Experiment with various materials to protect your sensitive skin and maximize your functional use of these areas. For your feet, try socks for diabetics, which do not have seams. For your arms, try covering your skin with similar soft socks with the toes cut off. When I could not bear the pressure of resting my burning, skinny elbows directly on my bed at night, I used to wrap my hands and elbows in stretched-out, cotton-polyester pillow fill bought in a roll at a fabric store. This allowed them to "float" and shifted the pressure considerably.

In addition, keep tabs on your skin's sensitivity level and try reducing it when you're feeling strong. You can use chenille washcloths to hold or slightly rub against your skin, or you can try sticking your hands or feet into containers of different textures, such as rice, water, and sugar.

Stay Independent with Mobility and Public Transport Services

If you're not able to drive yourself or walk by yourself to your medical appointments or other destinations, relying on the goodwill of your friends and family can become too much at times. Salvage some independence by utilizing your local transportation authority's paratransit/mobility services. With a note from your doctor stating your disability, you can receive pick-up and drop-off transportation in most states either free of charge or for the cost of a bus ride. The freedom of simply being able to go somewhere by yourself and make an appointment on your *own* time will be a treasured relief and will bolster your sense of independence. For more personalized services, see if a college student in your area would be willing to drive you to a few destinations per week for an hourly rate and the cost of gas; ask around for a trusted student or see if someone can post a notice at the local college or bookstore. Every once in awhile, go somewhere for pleasure rather than completing a chore or going to a doctor. Savor this time—you deserve it!

Another option for those with upper-extremity CRPS is to consider moving to a metro-and-bus-accessible location to drastically reduce your need to drive. I made this decision and am thankful for it, as six years passed before I could get back behind the wheel without it taking a significant toll on my body. Now I plan recuperation time for necessary drives and otherwise use public transport. Living near quality public city transport has kept me more easily connected to the outside world and my social support network, and has greatly reduced the constant demands placed on my arms.

Retrofit Your Car

If you are ready to drive yourself, there is an abundance of services waiting to ease you back behind the wheel. Adaptive driving companies offer electronic and structural adjustments for your vehicle that cater to your specific challenges and strength levels. If you have problems with your legs, electronic hand controls and wheelchair accessibility can be added to your vehicle. Likewise, "zero-effort steering" can reduce the amount of force required for painful arms to turn the steering wheel, and steering wheel knobs enable you to grasp the wheel with one hand. Finally, you can now electronically open your car door and turn on the engine with a key chain device. You may want to start with a driving evaluation given by a mobility specialist or your local hospital's adaptive driving department to pinpoint your specific needs and work with the car retrofitter. Personally, I regained the ability to drive by switching to a '98 Buick, as older American cars' steering wheels are often looser and easier to turn than newer varieties.

Be Careful with Overcompensating

When one part of your body is out of commission, the logical solution would be for other parts of your body to pick up the slack. Be careful with this! Overcompensating with one arm, leg, or other specific joints or muscles can quickly lead to additional injuries. In my experience, the injury of one hand led to overuse of the other.

Later, when I was unable to put on and tie my tennis shoes because both hands were so painful, I walked around my home barefoot for many months, which then led to painful nerve entrapments in each ankle. I also tended to use my legs extensively for getting up from the floor, opening the refrigerator door, and so on—eventually causing overuse of my knees.

The domino effect is a very real possibility that can last well into—and beyond—your experience with CRPS. The chain reaction of neuron hypersensitivity is a prominent and perplexing feature of this condition, so remember that you need every unaffected body part and cannot afford to carry more health problems than you've already been dealt. I practice what I call "spinning plates": incorporating as many forms of activity and body usage as possible so that when one movement feels risky, I just lay off and rely on another one for a little while. Along with this practice comes an assortment of braces and splints that I constantly change, depending on the activity involved; I remain vigilant about not resting one area too much and overusing another. Treasure these healthy parts, be aware of their vulnerabilities, and always keep an eye out for ways that you can encourage interaction and coordination of all body parts in your movement.

Nurture Yourself with Healthy Eating and Sufficient Sleep

Your body is a new being these days—one that is extremely sensitive to things you might not have thought twice about before. Don't push yourself on light sleep or meager foods, as your body needs adequate sleep and wholesome foods to heal. Nourish yourself with balanced meals; avoid sweets, caffeine, food with nitrates, alcohol, and overeating, which can send your body out of balance. Drink more water than you can even fathom, imagining how it maintains flow and circulation to all your needy tissues. Following Chinese medical wisdom imparted by my acupuncturist, I changed my meat-eating habits from intermittent meat eating to consciously ensuring that I ate a moderate amount of meat weekly to support nerve fiber myelination.

Support Your System with Supplements

Much recent coverage of supplements and their lack of regulation in the United States leaves this field wide open for varying perspectives. Talk with your doctor about trying a solid daily vitamin, along with a calcium supplement, vitamin E (200 to 400 IU), magnesium, fish oil, and possibly a glucosamine chondroitin sulfate complex. (Make sure both the glucosamine and chondroitin are sulfate complexes.) Not only does your body need extra support, but the prescription medications you're taking can deplete your body of certain nutrients at higher rates worth reviewing with a medical professional. Calcium is crucial, as CRPS does cause osteoporosis. Some patients and physical therapists have cited magnesium for aiding with muscular pain. Likewise, fish oil contains anti-inflammatory properties as a source of omega-3 vitamins. Finally, if you need to have a procedure or encounter another physical trauma, taking vitamin C has shown prophylactic properties against CRPS and should be considered. Talk with your doctor about any B vitamin needs she or he may consider for improving nerve function; B vitamin levels, dosage, and administration must be monitored carefully to ensure you do not take too much, as they can actually cause toxic nerve damage. In all cases, stay clear from megadoses of any vitamins and make sure that nothing interacts with your pharmacological regimen; the goal in systems support is balance and homeostasis. Super-high doses of supplements can be harmful or excreted uselessly.

You may want to consult with a specialist in homeopathic medicine and nutrition to tailor the use of natural substances to your personal mental-emotional-physical needs. However, you must be very careful to ensure that a natural substance you take does not cause a reaction with a pharmaceutical drug you're taking; both naturally occurring and synthetically produced substances or pills are very potent! Always check with your doctor and your homeo-pathic practitioner about interactions with any medication you are taking, along with proper dosage tailored to your needs.

Read Medical Information about CRPS
Only at "Safe" Times

CRPS medical resources, and even online patient sites, can seem so grave, so overwhelming, and so full of potential doom that you should select a time when you feel calm and detached enough to read about your condition. Put yourself in a place where you can keep perspective. Don't linger online before bedtime; you can save yourself added anxiety and pain by avoiding stirring up your nervous system via the worst-case-scenario fears and "what-ifs" that are generated by uncertain medical prognoses. Remember: Just as much as you can follow the path of a "horror story," so too can you turn in the opposite direction and improve. Go to sleep resting in the favor of positive probabilities and not the worst-case scenario. You need good sleep, and you need to nurture calm.

Sign Up with Medic Alert

For peace of mind and to ensure that hospital staff members address your special needs in case of emergency, register with Medic-Alert and include your CRPS information. MedicAlert Foundation is a nonprofit emergency medical information service that provides your data and directions on how to treat you to emergency room staff. You can avoid receiving venipuncture (surgical puncture of a vein for the purpose of drawing blood or inserting an IV) in painful areas, and if you need surgery, doctors know that they must proceed in a way that minimizes postsurgical CRPS flare-ups and spreading. When you sign up at www.medicalert.org or by calling (800) 432-5378, the organization records important contact information and treatment restrictions, and you receive a Medic-Alert bracelet to wear at all times.

Quick Pick-Me-Ups, Calmer-Downers, and Visualizations

Few people have gone through life unscathed by the memory of a few hours of acute pain. Yet what happens when pain becomes chronic, and—unlike the case with acute pain—there is no specific injury still causing it? Not only does CRPS hurt, but its alarming pain can be scary and demoralizing. It's important to know that your health can be affected by your reaction to this pain, and *every effort you can make to maintain inner balance and a positive spirit is an exercise in actual therapy.*

Rather than approaching your state of pain as an emergency, as one would in the case of typical acute pain, you will need to begin accepting the pain as a weight to bear indefinitely. Learn and practice mental techniques to support you in this task. This ability does not happen overnight, and it poses an ongoing challenge as long as pain exists—but you can make significant progress and take back control through this route. It is then that you will notice the interplay of emotions with your pain levels and some healing has an opportunity to start. It is a medical fact that CRPS interferes directly with your brain's experience of pain, emotion, and memory. Indeed, for the sake of wellness, your efforts to focus on positive ideas are ten times more important than the questions you want to ask about your pain.

When your spirit is beaten down and you need to reclaim this necessary balance of self, the following exercises can help in replenishing your spirit, releasing tense energy, comforting your soul and rethinking yourself. Take a deep breath and try one of these refreshers to remove your pain from the foreground. Then start over with your day until you hit the next hurdle.

Replenishing Your Spirit

Turn on the shower, sit down on the floor facing the faucet, and let a warm stream of water rain down on you as you pull your knees to your chest and rest your head over them. Close your eyes, focusing on the soothing, smooth quality of the water as it flows over you and trickles off your head. Imagine every inch of your painful spots being reached, purified, and washed away by the water's healing effect. Just five minutes of visualization and "shutting off" your mind and body can calm and refresh you.

Drink a glass of water, visualizing its purifying effect as it hydrates and adds flow within your tense body. Pay attention to its clarity as it spills over your tongue and travels down your throat, imagining its nourishing, life-giving liquid washing away toxins. Visualize it cooling your inflamed pain and loosening your stiff joints, tendons, and muscles. Concentrate on how necessary water is to optimizing your health and how therapeutic your gift of water to your body is at this time.

Find a gentle yoga video (via DVD or YouTube) that you enjoy and submit your mind and body to its movements when your nerve endings are acting up. Don't worry about ignoring your pain or shutting off your mind; the gentlest forms of yoga provide meditation *through* the movements, so your distress and pain will quiet and move to the background as you let yourself be carried along by the tape—and it takes time. Like taking a pill or using a medical procedure, remember that simply participating in yoga is a therapeutic act, so there is no need to clutter your mind with notions of what poses you can or cannot do. Congratulate yourself and mark your progress in the number of poses you can perform over time. Just one or two poses means progress!

I always do yoga at home, in a modified fashion for my needs. When I first started doing it, I used the video *Seated Yoga*. At first I could barely follow the instructions beyond one or two movements. However, I stuck to it, just for the simple idea that I was doing something good for my body—which gave me a better sense of peace and control in my treatment. In Chapter 6 you'll find a list of recommended yoga videos as well as further discussion of the benefits of yoga. Videos make it easier for you to stick to your commitment to do yoga frequently, and I've found that video instructors often seem more injury conscious than do yoga teachers at your local health club.

Releasing Energy and Frustration

If you used to handle frustration by doing something active or athletic, you'll notice that CRPS changes the options available for you to outwardly eliminate stress. Find the power and force of what you have inside that needs to be released and use this opportunity to take a closer look at it. Consider the alternative ways this book offers for channeling it.

Fill the sink with lukewarm water, stick your face in it, and blow bubbles. Scream, sigh out, release anxiety and frustration, and exhaust yourself through your blowing.

Music touches your spirit with sound. Pick a song that speaks to your mood—steering clear of quick beats—and sway gently along with it. Select something that is not so hyper that it makes you want to dance jerkily or release extra energy. Express yourself through its sound. Sing at the top of your lungs or breathe in profoundly, using your diaphragm to resonate deeply and release extra energy as you hum. Sometimes just one song can provide the time you need to release negative emotional toxins.

Express yourself, your sensations, and your angers by writing (or better by talking on voice-activated software). Release your emotions into words, let them become their own written entity, and let it all go. Your heightened sensitivity might have turned you into a poet! If writing isn't your style, try speaking your fears and concerns into a portable tape recorder; when you stop the tape, let them go for the day.

When pain and frustration would boil over, I used to sit in front of my computer and release my rage and questions onto the screen. The idea of writing this book also kept me sane at night and gave me a motivation and sense of meaning for staying so conscious of the pains, mistakes, and "bad breaks" that I seemed to be repeatedly experiencing. I began applauding myself for the little tricks and discoveries I made to treat myself, and I visualized the people I could help by sharing knowledge gained in my own trial by fire.

Laugh! Yes, it's hard to do with so much pain, but with a little help you can muster up one belly-laugh that can tighten and release your stomach muscles, draining tension. Flip on Comedy Central, Netflix, or a comedy show for a half hour, or better yet, watch stand-up comedy; with its rapid-fire jokes, it offers instant gratification and helps to drown out negative thoughts immediately. During my most intense early months of CRPS pain, I watched stand-up comics for hours at a time, blocking out worries and panic in focused desperation. Nowadays, I keep comedy close by for times when I want to continue an activity but physically cannot. Rather than fighting or lamenting my limitations, I shut off and change gears, resting my body during the transition. The *Jewish Comedy* channel on Pandora.com is a favorite on my smartphone.

Go outside and cry while it's raining. Connect your sorrows with nature, releasing them into the air, while being embraced by grander forces. Let the rain unite with and flood away your tears until you find calm again.

Try the following breathing technique: Lie on your back, breathe in for four counts, hold your breath for four counts, and breathe out for four counts. Focus on filling your stomach with your breath, rather than your chest—and watch your stomach rise up and down as you count. Visualize positive oxygen and health entering your body as you inhale and the release of negative energy, stale air, and the day's pains as you exhale in a smooth, controlled rhythm. Continue for twenty breaths.

Comforting Your Soul

Talk to the body parts that are hurting you. Develop a dialogue with them, expressing your frustrations—and your hopes. It may seem silly at first, but being able to direct these thoughts and feelings to where they most matter might make you feel better at times than telling a loved one. If you can bear the contact, kiss that body part or hug it against you as you build this connection while imagining blood flowing to the area and increasing circulation and healthy flow.

Get yourself a little stuffed animal, just a small one. Sound crazy? No mature adult is ever prepared for CRPS. Hold on to it or tuck it in your shirt on difficult afternoons or nights. It will provide extra comfort to your sensitive spirit and be a loyal companion during your minute-to-minute woes. It can be your little secret (like my stuffed lamb—and I was never attached to a stuffed animal as a child!).

Warm up a heating pad (whether homemade or store-bought), lie on your back, and place it over your chest. Concentrate on filling your chest with nurturing warmth and feeling grounded or secured by the extra weight. When heat permeates the chest, it can offer a deep sense of calm and sleepiness. The comfort of this position can lead you to a catnap or help you get to sleep at night. My sleep positions have often been limited to my back since I developed CRPS, and yet I crave the comfort of sleeping on my belly. I've found that placing a pillow on your chest while lying on your back can help you to feel grounded and comforted.

Go to a religious service that is familiar to you, even if you are not currently affiliated with a religion. The old rituals and songs from your childhood may soothe you and stir parts of yourself that you have not seen for a while. Singing other childhood songs, jingles, or camp cheers serves the same purpose. Involve your family and friends in singing sessions and tap this source of comforting familiarity and connection.

Walk or wheel yourself into the sun for a short spell, even if you don't feel like it. Focus on the warmth and light and contemplate yourself as closer to these natural forces. Feel the sun warming you through to your inner core, nourishing it, and reawakening your positive energy and earnestness. Watch for a tree blowing in the wind and imagine how you too can bend gracefully with the life challenges blowing your way.

Rethinking Yourself

This last part, rethinking yourself, is a biggie. Nerve pain, even just a nerve discomfort, can make you absolutely crazy. Use it! Claim it. If CRPS is going to set you apart from others, seize the difference. Claim the liberation of refusing to compare your sensations, dress, routine, adaptive aids, life, occupation, and character with those of everyone else. You face an ongoing challenge: to reframe your personality as something dynamic and grand enough to contain your abnormal physical sensations and altered perspective.

I look at it like this: When it comes to our personal lives, some of us like to think out-of-the-box, and some of us don't. Inside the box, everything is conventional and known and comfortable; outside, everything is unknown, exposed, or uncertain. The thing is, CRPS has just jumped into your box, making it stifling for you to live in there. CRPS is filling the place up, pushing you into corners, making it harder to breathe and function within the old limits and expectations of the pre-CRPS box. So, like it or not, you're going to have to break out of it if you want to live more comfortably. Open a window, stick a foot outside, take it slow, but realize there is a life outside of that box of hopes, values, and associations you've had all these years.

I often find myself losing perspective and forgetting that I will only be disappointed if I stick to the old-box thinking. Windows slam shut, and I constantly have to reopen them. Sometimes, when I'm feeling consistently well, I rush back inside and reclaim my old hopes and demands for optimal functional abilities again. I want to be back in the box, just like everyone else, with the same expectations in life—ones that do not involve CRPS. But then something happens—my hands start burning, and I am forced to face my physical limits again. I then have to pass through a bit of pain when I realize I have to reset my perspective to better fit my comfort zone.

Here are a few ideas to try for this rethinking process:

- Marvel at your body's ability to learn things in a new way. If your dominant hand is affected, train your other hand to write and complete other tasks. Dial the phone with your toes, master the recent explosion in smartphone voice-control features, and spare your hands. Introduce yourself to the new, different you, and throw away brain chatter about how you "used to" do things.

- If all your self-talk is irritated, spent, and linked to the triggers of pain and loss, step outside of your head temporarily by learning a new language. Whether it is a language you have always thought beautiful, one that evokes memories of a trip, or the language of your ancestors, sets of educational books and tapes are available for virtually any language at bookstores or the library. These sets offer refuge in a completely new and distant world of unintelligible sounds. You'll also discover a new angle on yourself.

  As soon as I could handle turning the pages of my father's old French book, I spent time each day pushing myself to absorb something completely different and beautiful through language. Waiting for my endless therapy visits, I kept a Walkman and French audiotape handy so that my "wasted" or "helpless" time was a chance to learn a new language. I also honored my roots and finally figured out the Yiddish words my grandparents had spoken to me since childhood by carrying a Yiddish audiotape with me for months.

- To nurture positive thinking, talk to yourself. As much as I have tried to eliminate negative thinking, I find that I cannot so easily dismiss or toss away worries, fears, and pessimism completely, but rather that I do well finding a limited space in which to isolate them. Outwit the voice and put it in its place!

  Unless you have a prior problem with multiple personality disorder, giving a name to the voice can help you make the distinction between yourself and the negative thoughts.

At my worst, I still entertained worries and negative thoughts daily, but I kept them separate from my core "Elena" self by associating that negative voice with another name. (I named mine Genevieve, although I don't know why.) Negative thoughts were Genevieve's jurisdiction, and I, Elena, could then get on with my day.

- Stick a temporary tattoo on an unaffected part of your body and feel whimsical and silly—even sexy—again. Focus on these parts as positive little secrets and experiment with what you or your partner defines as "sexy."

- Within the first few months of my struggle with CRPS, a good friend of mine created a T-shirt for me that said "I Am Sexy and Hands-Free" across the chest. What a great laugh that was! Beyond being a timely gift, this shirt is something I put on when I want to invite my playful side to come out for a few hours.

- Learn to forgive yourself. Since my CRPS developed from repetitive stress injuries, I am used to being someone who works hard; when I overdo it and then hurt, I blame myself harshly. As you learn to set new limits for your activity, your pain threshold can change from day to day. If you've become excited, wanted to embrace life more than you should have, and suffered the consequences, let it go. You know now that you have to rest, and you know your nerves will calm down once again. This is a learning process; you cannot possibly know how your body will react every moment.

- Remember that you are an innately pleasant and patient soul. Of course, nerve pain can make you irritable and edgy. It doesn't mean that you are a bad or unpleasant person. If you've lost your temper, think of all the women in labor and men in wartime who scream and bark at others while in pain. Dust yourself off, forgive yourself, and envision your "center of strength" for keeping calm next time.

♦ Cut the reel of your story leading up to CRPS that can play over and over in the search for faults and regrets. The time you waste on negative memories is time that places stress on your entire system. It is a cycle that never stops, and you are only winding yourself up. Consider a natural disaster and find your place within the bigger picture of life's whims and turns. Now consider all the uncertainty and possibilities of the future.

♦ Run through the new discoveries you've made about a friend or loved one since your diagnosis. Think of things you never knew before about him or her and what you'd still like to know. Now do the same, only about yourself.

Allison's story illustrates the power of using new, positive thought patterns to control pain through biofeedback, a complementary medical therapy. You'll learn more about this treatment modality in Chapter 6, "A World of Support: Complementary Therapies."

Allison's Story

I developed RSD after an auto accident in December 1989. I was rear-ended at less than five miles per hour but suffered whiplash nonetheless. For five solid years, I suffered the effects of global RSD, with unremitting, burning headaches and neck and shoulder pain as my chief complaints. At one point four years after the accident, I was seeing a neurologist who prescribed hard-core pain meds and antidepressants (for their off-label serotonin effects). His nurse called me one day and told me the doctor no longer wanted to treat me. I was offended and hurt, but that phone call became the turning point in my road to recovery.

At that moment, I went cold turkey off my meds and made the conscious decision that I would control my pain with the power of positive thought. I decided that Excedrin would be all I needed to take to help with the headaches. Within a year and a half, I went from having debilitating migrainelike headaches a minimum of five days per week to only a handful a month. I developed the ability to control my pain simply by meditating and concentrating it away.

My life returned to a relative state of normalcy, with the exception of having to accept some limitations surrounding my activities of daily living.

In May of 1998 I was rear-ended again, this time much more severely, resulting in a traumatic brain injury (among others) and an exacerbation of the RSD/CRPS symptoms. This time I was on total disability for seven months, and the pain was hovering around five to nine on the Leikert scale of one to ten. I was on Percocet, Vicodin, Soma, etc. to control the pain, but nothing helped. I took something for the pain every two hours, and I was lucky if it dropped by two to three points on the scale. Anything above a five was debilitating for me. Fortunately, one of my doctors knew of a PhD who practiced neurofeedback therapy. Neurofeedback is a form of biofeedback in which electrodes are placed on the head to record the brain's activity and determine how well the brain is functioning. Less than optimal brain wave patterns can cause sleep problems, mood/behavior problems, and decrease the body's ability to modulate pain, to name only a few. Once a patient is hooked up to the machine, he or she learns how to play computer games, using the mind as the joystick. The ability to successfully play a game is based on the patient's ability to control her brain wave patterns and focus her thoughts. It is an amazingly powerful tool and easy to master. I became proficient in a short period of time and was able to essentially go off the pain meds, again cold turkey. I realized this was a very similar therapy to what I'd taught myself to do years before.

Neurofeedback *literally* saved my life. I was so despondent and pain-ridden that I could not function and was downright suicidal. Learning how to regulate my own brain and its perception of the pain signals was profound—and remains equally profound to this day. Not only was I reasonably pain-free, but neurofeedback reinforced my positive outlook on life and perception that the human brain is an amazing and still relatively untapped resource for modulating the body's pain signals.

When I answer, "I'm fabulous! Wonderful! How are you?" whenever someone asks me how I am doing, I affirm the fact that I can play a very influential role in my body's health. Just because some doctor has given me a diagnosis of XYZ, I never claim ownership of that diagnosis. I guard my thoughts very carefully, and I live with the perception that only positive things are going to happen to me from now on.

Was this whole road to recovery easy? Goodness, no. It has been nearly fourteen years since I was first diagnosed with RSD and more than five years since the very debilitating accident in 1998. I am now a nationally board-certified and state-licensed acupuncturist and Chinese herbalist who specializes in pain management. I plan to go on to get a doctorate in either neuroscience or public health. Had I not truly embraced the idea of positive thought, I am nearly certain I would not be where I am today, both professionally and personally.

❖ ❖ ❖

At the root of all of these modifications and methods is the fact that you must undertake a major change in your activities and thoughts. You are a different person than you were before CRPS, and even a miraculous elimination of all pain will not return you to exactly who you were previously. It is normal and necessary that you pass through the process of grieving for your old self. It is also required that you make a new "blueprint" of yourself and invite adaptive ways into its creation.

For example, with CRPS, I've become a jack-of-all-trades in many areas I never knew existed. I'm a master meteorologist, able to detect when it's going to rain within an hour or stop raining within two because my pain levels rise and ease with the subtle change in barometric pressure. I'm a colorful analogy maker, endlessly painting conceptual images so others can understand my body sensations and worries about the future. I can help others with obscure neurological complaints, as I have spent so much time researching the extended circle of CRPS-related conditions. I can spell words out loud in a split second, after years of using voice-activated software.

Well before I returned to regular full-time work, I served as a Spanish medical translator for a few hours per week for a local charity and then a hospital, as a way to feel useful without returning to hand-demanding work. It provided a new mental challenge that I never would have taken on if I did not need to drastically reconsider my future life path due to CRPS; I'd had to leave my career as a communications writer. I found I was a better, more empathetic volunteer, knowing all too well the patients' need for company or adaptive equipment that would allow them to function on their own.

Gathering your own lessons learned and taking stock of your new, added abilities or personality traits is a crucial way to set you on your path toward healing, a new lifestyle, and maybe even a new career. These things come slowly, creeping forward and sometimes pulling back as your optimism and "good days" struggle with physical setbacks and lost hopes. It's important to start small and not to put yourself under pressure to do this "right."

Moreover, coming to terms with your limitations doesn't rule out breakthrough grieving moments later on. It is a constant, conscious campaign to decide how you will react to your physical barriers and decide, eventually, when giving in to the grief is necessary and when it doesn't serve you. Sometimes these decisions are made every hour on the hour, in response to specific pain levels or restricted activities. Keep pushing forward!

On a smaller scale, remember how you can convert a painful hour, day, or general state into something productive or meaningful, directing your attention to the gains rather than the losses of this experience. The trick will be in expanding your definition of what is personally "productive" or "meaningful" to you. For me, the extra time during which I have been physically limited has made an opportunity to connect more with my family and friends. Some friendships have suffered since CRPS, but others have deepened. Oftentimes when I don't feel like talking about my woes, the silence I give to a friend allows him or her to enjoy me as a better listener. Feeling bad? Pick up the phone and build a deeper relationship with a loved one. This, too, is an accomplishment. Or rather than lament the loss of things you used to like to do, find something for which you might not have had patience before—such as listening to classical music, meditating, sketching, taxidermy, reading, your child's science homework, and so on. This is your opportunity to take a closer look at things around you, and by focusing so closely, you can mentally push at least some of your pain to the background.

As you move through this personal transformation, the next two chapters consist of interviews with experts who can guide you.

Direct from the Practitioner: A Conversation with a Physician

It's true that you'll have to become a bit of your own "expert" on CRPS, keeping up-to-date on clinical research and articles from informed organizations such as associations. However, a good practitioner offers an unmatched personal element, which is essential to your care. Finding a practitioner who extends trust, understands your condition, and envisions a broad treatment and lifestyle strategy can help you regain a sense of control. Power begins with applying teachings from the doctor's office to your life at home.

What are your doctors' and therapists' philosophies towards CRPS treatment? Seeing this bigger picture through their eyes can help you map out your place within the CRPS maze, clearing up some questions and tangents along the way. In fact, an inside look into your doctor's or therapist's approach can also assist you in ironing out bumps along the road that might occur regarding new treatments or therapeutic modalities with which he or she might not be familiar or comfortable. While being treated by an expert on the forefront of CRPS research would be the ideal for any patient, this is simply not the reality for most. It is important to talk with as many professionals as possible in order to prepare yourself for dialogue with your doctor and therapist. This chapter and the next consist of interviews with two practitioners who lend their insights into very different aspects of clinical treatment of CRPS and the whole person who comes with it.

We begin with Dr. Edward Carden, a caring anesthesiologist and interventional pain-management specialist who has treated hundreds of CRPS patients. Having a loved one with CRPS initially drew Carden into the disease's realm of challenges. Representing the wisdom of conventional Western medicine and the role of a doctor for your care, he shares with you his viewpoints on CRPS treatment and expectations of your doctor.

An Interview with Edward Carden, MD, FRCPC, FACA, DipAAPM

Dr. Edward Carden is a retired clinical professor at the University of Southern California Keck School of Medicine, and at present the director of Southern California Academic Pain Management and the director of the Southern California Reflex Sympathetic Dystrophy Institute. A diplomate member of the American Academy of Pain Management, he is also a member of the Royal College of Physicians of Canada.

As a treating physician, how would you define CRPS?
There are certain guidelines that are used for the definition of RSD, the name of which was changed in 1994 to *complex regional pain syndrome*. However, from my perspective as a treating physician, anybody who's got pain out of proportion to the injury, pain that has any of the *sequelae* [pathological, secondary consequences resulting from a primary condition] of CRPS and the cause cannot be ascertained, has CRPS until proven otherwise. CRPS is a condition that usually occurs peripherally in the body, which means an arm or a leg, and the distribution of the pain is in a glove or stockinglike pattern. There should be—although in my experience, all these features are not necessarily present—pain that is usually

burning. There is often shooting pain. There is often swelling and heat in the early stages of the disease and cooling in the late stages of the disease. There are abnormalities of function with progressive weakness, and there's often inability to use the particular extremity because of pain.

Basically, the normal way you want to define CRPS is loss of function, change in sympathetic tone (i.e., heat, sweating, or coldness), and pain, which is usually burning. Another factor is that there is usually hypersensitivity of the skin, called allodynia, in which you might just touch the skin and experience excruciating pain. All this occurs after what may be a trivial injury, or in some cases, no injury at all.

Not all of the symptoms are always present. As a practicing physician, I don't care how many the patient has. So it would seem that the purists will define CRPS in a certain way, requiring a certain number of these symptoms to make the diagnosis, whereas a treating physician will define it somewhat differently, usually by using the response to a sympathetic block as the deciding factor.

The most important thing from my point of view—certainly in early cases—is how the patient responds to sympathetic block correctly delivered, and that is the most important thing.

How many patients with CRPS have you treated over the years?
Six hundred or so; I don't know exactly.

How did you get exposed to or involved in CRPS treatment?
I'd see an occasional article on CRPS in anesthesia journals. They'd suggest doing a stellate ganglion block [an upper-extremity sympathetic block] if you suspected a patient had CRPS in the upper extremity. So years ago I'd have the odd patient roll in, and I started doing blocks if I thought she or he had CRPS. When I'd do them, the pain would go away—but it would come back after a (very) variable length of time. Then I'd say to myself, "Now what the heck do I do?" So I started calling people who were "experts" to try to find out.

At that point, I had a friend who developed CRPS in the shoulder. I shipped this patient off to top-rated experts for treatment. They didn't seem to be improving the condition! So I went all over the place—I went to Europe, I went all over America—to find out how best to treat it. And in doing that, I worked out my own way of treating it, based on the best I found from them.

How do you explain the mechanism of pain in CRPS to a patient?
The theory that best fits—or at least simplifies—all the knowledge we have so far is as follows. Indeed, what we have is a problem with hyperexcitability of what they call wide dynamic range neurons in the spinal cord. Those nerves are in the dorsal horn, where the nerves first run in from the periphery to the spinal cord. They are sending messages to the brain saying, "There is pain here." The brain responds by telling the patient that they have pain. A-beta nerve [touch] fibers normally send messages through at a constant rate of firing to these wide dynamic range neurons. If you decrease the epinephrine around these fibers by doing a sympathetic block, the rate at which they fire drops right off, the wide dynamic range neurons cease to be hyperexcitable, and the pain goes away.

So if you take someone who has CRPS and you inject epinephrine, the pain goes up. If you do a sympathetic block, the pain goes down. That's the theory, which the majority of experts subscribe to because it fits perfectly with what you see.

What is your take on the other theories regarding the CRPS mechanism, the ones that say it is based on inflammation or free radicals?
Let me say that there are obviously other elements involved in this, such as immune system dysfunction and central nervous system disease. The theory that I've seen personally, which fits with what we know and see clinically, is the one that I have given you. That's the one that most experts stick to at this time with most treatment strategies. There are certainly additions to that, but I'd prefer to steer away from the complexity of research observations until we know more.

If you want, you can look at it this way: Imagine that you run into a brick wall and smash your knee against the wall. It's painful. Now, your body sends information to the spinal cord indicating that "this knee was just smashed against a wall." And it hurts. So what does your body do? It increases blood flow to the area. It will swell and will get hot, angry, and very painful to walk on for awhile. That is the body's response to an injury: stop the motion in the area, increase the blood flow to the area, and create swelling. You'll also have pain, so you won't use it. The body can then heal itself, and all those symptoms go away.

With CRPS, it never goes away. The body thinks there's something wrong there because injury messages are going to the brain, causing the body to continue the pain, continue the muscle spasm going on in the area so you cannot use it, and continue to have the blood flow in, creating swelling and heat. Then after a while, you get "burnout" of the spinal cord. As to theories about this, either the body says, "Hey, the heat business didn't work. Why don't we try making it cold?" Or the other theory is you have damage to the central nervous system. This changes the sympathetic flow to the area, and the affected area suddenly switches from being hot and swollen to being cold, clammy, and sweaty.

Let's consider this idea of CRPS transitioning from being peripheral to becoming centralized in the brain. Is this what you call the centralized transition?
Sure, that is what you could call centralized. That's when it's more difficult to treat, because you know that you've got changes in the body going on, creating an almost irreversible state. Do note that the original theories about there being four stages of CRPS can really be thrown out now. The originator of the theory based it on the patients a physician saw in a few cases, so he wrote them up many years ago and it stuck. I've seen lots of people come in who have not progressed like he stated and who did not follow the classic stages at all. Everyone is different.

What is your normal treatment method?

My main four components for treatment are blocks, physical therapy, medications, and psychotherapy. [For a discussion of the role
of psychotherapy in the treatment of RSD/CRPS, see Chapter 6, "A
World of Support: Complementary Therapies."] My methods are
specially tailored to be simple and effective. For example, when a
patient comes in with arm CRPS pain, I first do one stellate ganglion block because that is the standard. When that's done, and the
patient has a positive response, I will start doing brachial plexus
blocks (another regional sympathetic block), because they are far
less invasive. I use a 27-gauge needle, which is very small, and
the patient barely knows he's getting stuck. With stellate ganglion
blocks, there's a significant complication rate. Patients can get
hoarse, lose their voice, get bleeding and even esophageal perfora-
tion—all sorts of things—and they are unpleasant for the patients;
whereas interscalene blocks (a type of brachial plexus block) have
minimal complications. So sometimes I will regularly do twenty of
these blocks in patients, while the old theory stated to do five and
give up if the patient didn't get better.

*Speaking still of blocks, do you think there is a certain limiting factor
in how many blocks are too many?*

With CRPS, I don't limit blocks. If the patients are continuing to
improve, I will continue to do them—but I will make sure that the
block is something simple and not likely to cause complications.
Interscalene blocks are a good example. I have one patient who is
kept well and working full-time and functional by receiving weekly
blocks for years; it depends on what works for the patient, and our
remaining open to trying other options when blocks are not working. I suppose I should explain how I use the blocks.

Usually when a patient comes in during the early stages, I will
do a block that causes their pain to go away—and it comes back
after a certain length of time. It may be a day, two days, three days.
When the pain comes back, I ask the patient, "How is your pain

now?" And they will say, "It came back exactly the same as before," or the patient might say, "Less." Then, based on the answers, I split the patients up into different groups in terms of treatment tracks. With the patients who get decreasing pain after the block wears off, you keep blocking them, getting ever-decreasing pain levels until it's gone! With the patients whose pain returns the same but each block lasts longer and longer, you start reblocking before the effects of the previous block wear off and continue until the pain does not return, doing blocks at ever increasing intervals. In the meantime I have them doing physical therapy, taking appropriate medications, and seeing a pain psychologist, which is very necessary.

For patients who do not respond to blocks, what happens?
I repeat the sympathetic block a different way. I do a different type of sympathetic block, such as an epidural, brachial plexus, or intravenous regional block.

If the result is still negative, I assume that the patient doesn't have CRPS or has sympathetically independent pain (SIP). If it's SIP, treatment is physiotherapy, medications, and psychotherapy and likely ketamine. We look at options; sometimes it may instead be a spinal cord stimulator. With ketamine, I sometimes have the patient try an hour-long intravenous infusion and see what effect it has. If it's positive, I may put them on the ketamine pill, which is often covered by insurance more than infusions right now. So, we work again with a list of options. You have to be very careful with the pills, though, as people can get high off of them if they are broken apart and snorted. I've heard the same from some patients who have used the nasal spray, as one patient got high as a kite on his and asked to return the drug. This is an FDA-approved substance, but it's very powerful. I also work with patients to undergo a longer ketamine infusion treatment, and we see how that works.

If that doesn't work, we look at a spinal cord stimulator. And, if the spinal cord stimulator doesn't work, we consider an intrathecal pump that can deliver medication far more powerfully than medication taken orally. A pump might be used to deliver Dilaudid, and other drugs to help.

What is your approach to drug therapy?
CRPS is complicated, but I try to follow the KISS method: Keep It Simple, Stupid. I use a lot of logic in my treatment approaches. There are all sorts of new drugs coming out for neuropathic pain, but I still use a lot of Neurontin as the drug of choice. I also use phenoxybenzamine, which is an alpha sympathetic blocker. I base what I do on the results I have had with my patients.

You need different drugs for different things. Neurontin will usually take care of the basic pain of CRPS by helping with the burning and skin sensitivity—that's number one. Then for shooting pains, Tegretol helps. If you want to get rid of some of the basic pain, people oftentimes give Elavil. I keep away from Elavil for one basic reason, particularly in women: It makes them gain weight. Pamelor is a good substitute. Often a mood-enhancing drug, such as Paxil, is needed, as well as a good sleeping pill. We must not of course forget analgesics from aspirin to morphine. The patient must be kept as pain-free as possible.

You give people exactly what they need, and if they've got something specific, such as a cold hand or foot, I will give them phenoxybenzamine and/or Regitine, which is a sympathetic alpha-blocker. It treats the most basic problem by providing a sort of sympathetic block. I try to narrow down the pills so that there are only enough going in to deal with the specific problems they're facing. Sometimes I experiment and give a patient a "drug holiday"—take them off of what they are taking and then slowly put them back on again. Some patients do very well if they do that.

What about topical medications, such as topical ketamine?
I've seen mixed results in ketamine cream so far. I've seen clonidine patches have worked better for a focal site of pain. For example, you may have disperse pain in your hand, but if you can find a focal source for the pain, one-inch square patches should be put over

that area—and they usually help. Lidocaine patches will work in certain people if the real focal point of the pain source is close to the skin.

Does your treatment plan follow the same steps, usually?
No. I have guidelines, like I said, but we look at options. I want to explain further about the problems with blocks that patients might have. If the stellate ganglion block was done blindly, without fluoroscopic control [a method of following a block's path inside the body by continuously viewing shadowy images formed by the transmission of X rays through the area, appearing on a fluorescent screen], one doesn't really know where the drugs went except that someone stuck the needle down onto a piece of bone on the spine and injected the medication. In order to get CRPS in the arm under control, one needs to block the first, second, and third thoracic sympathetic ganglia, which lie in front of the T-1, -2, and -3 thoracic vertebral bodies. When one does a sympathetic block correctly, the medication will run down from the end of the needle, to the thoracic spine, and block the sympathetic ganglia. Then one gets the desired result, and the pain in the arm goes away.

So if the block is not done correctly—i.e., the needle doesn't get inserted into the direct tissue plane—the drugs will not run into the upper part of the chest, and the result will not be good. These blocks should always be done under X-ray control, with injection of dye first.

How can patients ensure that they receive the right type of block from a doctor?
That is always a problem. It's important to get a block from a recognized CRPS interventional pain-management specialist and not a neurologist, internist, chiropractor, or orthopedist. It's very difficult for patients to get through to their doctors, to get the doctors to do what they should, because a lot of doctors don't really know enough about treating the disease, so make sure you have the right doctor for the job. For instance, I just talked to a lady on the phone

who called up about her daughter. The daughter has CRPS. The daughter went to a pain center, they started to treat her, and they put an epidural catheter in her and took it out after three days. The treating physician said, "But we never do it for longer than this," and took it out. Now, people who really deal with this disease will run the catheter for three or four weeks, during which time the patient is in therapy and other modalities, which help the patient get better. Some brave doctors even keep the catheters in for up to six months.

I also think it's important to use a very small needle. I add a drug to my blocks that serves to reduce scar tissue, which is important, especially if you have repeat blocks.

At this point, I should mention for your readers something that will help them with treatment. CRPS 1 and 2—RSD and causalgia—have all the same symptoms and are basically the same disease, except with causalgia there is damage to a major nerve, and with CRPS there is often damage to a small nerve. So when I have a patient with CRPS, I still immediately look for the source of their pain. I'll do a sympathetic block so the pain goes away. Then I'll go into the area where the pain was coming from, and I'll tap the patient, which usually causes the patient to say, "Oh! I feel electricity running from here to there." That is a neuroma on the nerve. That is the source of the pain. That neuroma has been firing off ectopic impulses of the spinal cord, causing this disease. I will then destroy the neuroma. I can freeze it or use radiofrequency or phenyl. At this time, if one diagnoses the disease early, often one can cause an instant remission or cure the disease.

Destroying neuromas surgically instead can be a real problem. This is what I argue about with my surgical colleagues, because if you take the end of a nerve and bury it—which is what surgeons do—and if the CRPS doesn't go away, the neuroma then grows in that location. Now you've got a real problem, and you've got to try to find it. Whereas, if I leave the nerve where it is and destroy the neuroma there, I know where it is. If the neuroma grows back, I can destroy it again next year.

I've got a great case history for you just to demonstrate the neu-roma theory. There were two brothers, both of whom had CRPS, both of whom had arthroscopies done—one to the shoulder, and one to the knee. Both had portal neuroma—the portal being where they stuck the scope in. When they stuck the arthroscope in, it hit a nerve, damaged the nerve, and the nerve developed a little neu-roma that sparked the CRPS. I destroyed the neuromas, and both of these men are fine.

I have to say, I have gone to big meetings with researchers from all over the place who did not buy the idea of nerve entrapments or neuromas being involved with CRPS cases. Yet if you look it up, there is an orthopedist by the name of Hungerford who wrote an article years ago in an orthopedic journal about a nerve that supplies the knee and runs down the inside of your leg, called the saphenous nerve. When they put a knee scope in, they go straight where that nerve is and can damage it. The article claimed that this causes CRPS. This is orthopedic literature from years ago—this is nothing new—but to get everybody else to believe it, it's amazing how difficult it is.

You see, most surgeons do not think about CRPS. It is rarely on their minds because the awareness was never there when they went to medical school. They were never taught about the disease.

Were you ever taught about it during your education?
When I was at medical school, I was taught minimally about it.

Is there a certification program as it stands, right now, for CRPS treatment?
There aren't any that I know of.

Has there ever been a time you've given a patient a block and for whatever reason, it did not work at all? Have you had patients who did not respond to blocks?
[Yes.] If I see patients who are a few years down the line with CRPS already, these are people with what is called sympathetically

independent pain. I've been talking mostly up to now about patients with sympathetically maintained pain, the ones who are usually in the early stages.

At what point do you find patients to be splitting into sympathetically maintained pain and sympathetically independent pain?
It varies very much, based on my experience. Sometimes it can be six months to a year, sometimes it can be five to six years. No two CRPS patients are the same.

Can you explain the difference between sympathetically maintained pain and sympathetically independent pain?
The theory is that the wide dynamic range neurons in the spinal cord are surrounded by other cells, some of which calm the neurons down when they are excited. Some of the calming down cells die off, so now you're never going to calm the neurons down and the effects of a sympathetic block do no good now. A lot of this stuff is theoretical but it makes sense. There are researchers who have created diseases similar to CRPS in rats and rabbits, then dissected the spines to derive this information.

Spreading is a great fear for many people with CRPS. Can you discuss this a little bit and explain how this happens?
Every patient is different. When it comes to spreading, the theory is that you have these excitable nerves in the spinal cord. They are lined up on top of each other, all the way up to the brain. So one fires up the next one above it, which fires the next one above that, which fires the next one up, and so on. There is this chain reaction in which more and more nerves get excitable. That's why if you have CRPS in the hand, for example, it spreads up the arm to the shoulder. And when, under treatment, it disappears, the pain usually leaves starting from the shoulder and moving down to the hand. It will normally spread up from an extremity toward the body.

Similarly, it can actually spread across the spinal cord to the other side. What is actually happening when you have CRPS is that you are being told you have pain by some nerves in your brain. And as more and more cells in the spinal cord keep getting excited, your brain will tell you that you've got more and more pain—which you do.

Because they have thrown out the idea of these strict stages for CRPS, do you think there is still a statistic proving the odds of CRPS spreading in someone? We have seen statistics on a 25 percent chance of spreading, and in other instances there is a 70 percent chance of spreading.
I would say that 25 percent is more to the mark.

Do you think it is possible to increase the quality of life dramatically in someone whose CRPS has progressed for a long period of time?
Absolutely.

What are the expectations that people in this situation can have, once they find the "right" treatment—albeit very late?
If they go to a good doctor who knows what he or she's doing, excellent. But if they go to the wrong person, then they're going to go down the other path. The whole trick is to read books like [this one] with the right references and look up what they should be doing or where they should go. In the late stages, you need an interested, caring doctor, an excellent physiotherapist, and lots of hard work—not forgetting a pain psychologist's help over the rough spots.

Patients need to call and ask around to find someone who is an invasive pain management specialist. There's an American Society of Interventional Pain Physicians, based in Kentucky, that patients can call to find someone in their area. This organization is a good start. Otherwise, there are doctors scattered around the country who really know what they're doing.

If people get onto the RSDSA website [www.rsds.org] and download a few articles, they should take them to their doctor and say "Look, this is what you should be doing." Maybe some of them will take notice. Every so often I'll get a phone call from an out-of-state doctor who says, "A patient just came in with this article. How do I do this, that, and the other?" and I'll explain.

For these types of patients—what can they expect when finally seeing the right doctor after so long? Being that not every patient does recover. I know that Cynthia Toussaint, the founder of For Grace [a women-in-pain advocacy organization], was one of your patients who dramatically moved back into life—after being originally rolled into your office on a gurney. Do you have case histories that you'd like to share?

By the time Cynthia came to me, she was fifteen years into untreated CRPS. She had true sympathetically independent pain. She is where she is now because she never gave up hope and she worked very, very hard to get back to an active life.

When I do get a patient who is way down the line, I do the same things that I've been telling you about. Sympathetic blocks if they still work, medication, physical therapy, not forgetting, of course, the psychotherapist. And ketamine. Then, if none of that is working, I try a spinal cord stimulator. This works in most cases. If I go ahead and put in a spinal cord stimulator that helps with the pain, sometimes dramatically, it can actually help wind down the CRPS. There have been a lot of case reports in which spinal cord stimulators have been put in, and after two or three years, patients got better.

How does this happen, theoretically?

Spinal cord stimulators create tingling in the mind instead of pain. This can, in fact, seemingly help to calm down these wide dynamic range neurons and slow things down. No one quite understands how all of this works; it just does! And the last thing you can do is try the intrathecal pump. The thing is, narcotics taken orally or even intravenously with CRPS do not work well against the pain. However, narcotics given intrathecally into the spine do. One puts a morphine pump in and you run the morphine, or whichever other narcotic you select into the spinal fluid, and combat the pain that way.

So for a patient who has the spinal cord stimulator perhaps on high, twenty-four hours per day, utilizing this is a good thing because it can actually help on an overtime basis to reduce hypersensitivity of the spinal cord nerves?

Yes. This has happened in patients, and while I cannot give you the number, it is relatively high. The new tendency is actually to put spinal cord stimulators in sooner rather than later. Unfortunately, this is a risk. There are too many doctors who might do one sympathetic ganglion block, and when it doesn't work, they advise putting in a spinal cord stimulator.

So you do disagree with putting in stimulators early?

Absolutely not that early! You must do all the basic treatment work first to try to get it under control. Physical therapy, blocks, and medication, etc., for at least a few months! If these are not working, then you put in an epidural infusion for at least three weeks, with therapy, to break the pain cycle. Then consider ketamine. Maybe you can consider putting a stimulator in. That, at least, is what I do.

In your papers, you also advocate physical therapy as a crucial component of treatment. Are there any times in which you might discourage physical therapy?

The most important thing with physical therapy is that you must do it correctly. The standard for physical therapy is isometric strengthening and passive range of motion. When I first started doing this, [physical therapists] used to mess up my patients, and they would come back worse. For example, I had a patient with CRPS in his knee, and he was put on an exercise bicycle and came back with more pain. If it's a knee problem, you can do whichever type of straight-leg raises you can find that does not irritate the problem area in your knee. The physical therapist, rather than the patient, then puts the knee passively through its full range of motion.

It is thought that ice is bad, and most patients—certainly in the early stages of CRPS—will jump if you put ice on them. Most of the time, heat will really help.

What is your view on sympathectomy?
Sympathectomy is another animal. A review article by Raja covering all previous articles on sympathectomy showed that 10 percent of sympathectomies done for various reasons have complications. The complication rate for sympathectomy done to treat neuropathic (i.e., CRPS) pain is 30 percent. A lot of these people can have a return of pain, and if they do, you can no longer do a sympathetic block to get rid of it. Then you've got these people in terrible pain that you cannot treat. And so in my book, surgical sympathectomy is out. I will occasionally do a radiofrequency sympathectomy in which you burn a piece of the sympathetic nerve, knowing that it will likely regrow—just to give the patient enough time to do physical therapy and start getting better. You've got to be very careful, and if you ever do attempt to do a surgical sympathectomy, you are mandated to sit down with a patient and say, "Look, we can do this for you. You may get cured, but you've got a 30 percent chance of being in pain, which is possibly worse because we have no way to treat it."

Now, you know radiofrequency sympathectomies can have their own complications as well.
Yes. But I only do a partial sympathectomy in the hope that it will "take the edge off"—and primarily just for CRPS located in the lower extremity because you don't want to destroy the stellate ganglia.

What you think is the most difficult or devastating thing you see in your patients with CRPS? How do you see it affect them psychologically?

For most patients, it's the lifestyle change. They are in constant pain, their family may shun them, and people don't want to know about them anymore. They have this enormous problem while everyone else thinks they are nuts. I have lines of patients coming in with the same story. This can cause big psychological problems. They can't do the sports they used to do, and so on, and so on.

What do you consider to be the relationship between the mind and pain, and how can patients use this knowledge to their advantage?
It is a very good question. First of all, this is not a psychiatric disease. The pain comes first, and then people risk getting bent out of shape because of it. As far as the mind controlling pain goes, biofeedback can be used very effectively. It's not going to cure these people, but it is very effective in helping them and lowering their pain levels. It is a good adjuvant to basic treatment. There are some studies that have been done claiming that they can get their pain levels down from a seven to a four with biofeedback, and I'm sure that's true.

Why is it that biofeedback works, especially in examining the case of someone whose pain has become centralized?
Biofeedback really is based, in my mind, on yoga. You're looking to control your own body—the subconscious parts of your body. With biofeedback, you are learning to control the input of pain to your brain. It's the same idea as hypnosis helping people to control the subconscious.

How do you advise your patients to prepare themselves for flare-ups or setbacks on their own?
My approach to patients is this: When they get here, first of all, they're mad at the world—mad at me, mad at everybody. They get the first sympathetic block on board, and they suddenly find the pain reduced. I will say to them, " Look, you're in a tunnel. At the end is a light, and you are heading there. The pain's going to go up and go down and go up and go down, with good days and bad days,

but overall we are going to get you better." That's the way I approach patients. If they understand it's going to get worse sometimes but overall it's going to be improving, patients are usually very happy with that. Because even when they have a flare-up, they can think, "Tomorrow I will be better."

While his specialty is clearly conventional medicine, Dr. Carden supports his patients' interests in trying other complementary therapies to enhance efforts in restoring function. Thus, it is important to remember that your doctor does not need to be an expert in both types of medicine—or even CRPS (though how nice would that be?). However, he or she *must be willing to continually learn about CRPS*, explore its treatment idiosyncrasies, support your integration of complementary modalities, and keep up-to-date on clinical information. You, in turn, can help him by apprising him or her of journal articles and updated materials that have been provided by reputable RSD/CRPS organizations.

Direct from the Practitioner: A Conversation with a Complementary Care Provider

Offering the "flip side" to the previous chapter's conventional medical specialty is Sheri Barnes, who specializes in the therapeutic aspects of acupuncture, massage, and occupational therapy. Her work is largely hands-on and highly personalized, providing the day-to-day pain relief and encouragement that is crucial to a CRPS patient's care. Together, the combination of these disciplines—Western and Eastern medicine, allopathic and alternative—can provide a multidisciplinary and holistic treatment plan, each aspect bestowing its own benefits and wisdom. In this chapter, Barnes explains acupuncture, as well as a new way to consider yourself in relation to your body in pain.

An Interview with Sheri Barnes, MAc, OTR/L

Sheri Barnes is a licensed occupational therapist, acupuncturist, and massage therapist with the Center for Occupational and Environmental Neurology in Baltimore, Maryland.

How do you define illness?
I define it as anything that invades your function, meaning that even the smallest sickness has now become lodged and become the central focus in your life in a very disruptive way. It may have

changed how you dress in the morning, how you think, and so on. It has started to become ever-present in your life, and you don't know how to stop it.

How would acupuncture principles approach the definition of disease?
The word *disease* includes "ease," which is almost like your birthright; that's the way our bodies are meant to function—in a state of homeostasis, in a state of balance. When that becomes dislodged, you have disease.

What happens to a person's body, mind, and spirit when that illness becomes chronic?
When an illness becomes chronic, you will see that the disruption of daily life will become somehow deeper. On a bodily level, it is always there—even when you go to sleep at night or wake in the morning. On a mental level, it invades almost your every thought, and on a spiritual level, it will almost prevent your ability to restore yourself. It beats you down, so that the part of you that says, "Well, tomorrow's another day"—the hope for tomorrow—can be missing.

What's the most crucial thing that enables patients to begin a path toward CRPS healing?
It's most important for you to search out and take back, if you will, that one part of you that is not invaded by this illness or injury, the one part of you that is whole and complete and well—even if it's just for this minute. It's important to recognize what's going well or what is well inside of you rather than always concerning yourself with what is not well. There's always the chance to look at how you are functioning and how you are being successful rather than how you're failing. That's very important.

How, in basic terms, does acupuncture work?
Acupuncture works with needles that are very strong stimuli. They change the way that your insides flow. Some people call that

chi, some people call that energy, but it's really the joining of that flow—blood flow, nervous flow, everything—that helps us be well and be able to heal ourselves.

These strong stimuli direct the energy in different ways, either from too much energy in one place or not enough energy in another, to cause a change in that "flow"—the flow of your body's abilities to heal itself. In my acupuncture treatment, getting rid of blockages or obstacles is most important.

There's also a substance called moxa, made of mugwort, that is used in conjunction with the needles. It's a substance that is burned on the skin without causing an actual burn to the skin, and it's very nourishing to the body.

Are there certain types of blockages that you, in particular, have seen in people with CRPS?
Every person is different. With some people with CRPS, I have gone right ahead and started moving energy around, but it's not been as successful as when I've looked to find where the blockages were and just aimed to remove them.

How exactly does acupuncture's change in flow affect pain reduction, anxiety control, and calming effects? How do these physical, mental, and emotional benefits go hand-in-hand?
Well, the fact that there are mental worries going on when your hand is aching all the time and doesn't work well is testament to the fact that there is a body-mind-spirit connection. Acupuncture works to restore all these levels. Going back to that theory of *disease,* if we can reduce the dysfunction or blockages or disharmony in that area of your body, then your mind and spirit will be replenished, and you'll be able to go on and think about other things.

How long does it take normally for acupuncture to provide relief? Is it a quick fix, or does it take time?
It's never wise to think of acupuncture as a quick fix, although people often will see immediate benefits from it and feel better right

after treatment. I tell people that six to ten treatments is a good trial, and if you or your practitioner is not seeing any benefits by that time, then I'd say it's time to try to another type of acupuncture or a different treatment modality.

You mentioned other types of acupuncture. What types are you talking about?
Well, there's a symptom-relief acupuncture, called medical acupuncture, where there's a medical prescription: You have a pain in your leg, therefore you get a prescription of particular needles to stick in your body to treat that leg. That's one kind of acupuncture, while the kind of acupuncture I practice gets more to the roots of the problem. If you take an example by using a tree, medical acupuncture might treat and repair the tree's limb; the kind of acupuncture I practice, called traditional five elements acupuncture, would treat its roots and assume everything else gets better after that step.

The thought of inserting needles into a painful limb seems scary to many CRPS patients. How would you work around a limb too painful to touch?
It is contraindicated to stick a needle into that limb or part of your body, so I would stick the needles into the other limb, or a hand, etc. It's important to know that the needles going in are not giving you anything or taking away anything, but they are in fact self-regulating, and they are tapping into a flow inside your body—a flow that you were born with and will die with. These needles are not foreign objects or prescriptive doses—they are rather tapping into something that is already there and encouraging something already inside you to adjust.

So you can still benefit one side of your body if you stick a needle into the other side, for example?
This is true. The surprising thing is it is often not necessary to perform the acupuncture in the area where the CRPS shows up.

Oftentimes people are very surprised when they are told to expose their backs to treat a flare-up in their arms. This does not mean the practitioner is avoiding the CRPS, but rather he or she is getting to the root and clearing toxins, blockages, and so on.

And whenever people have concerns about their acupuncture treatment, it's okay to talk with a practitioner about every acupuncture point. For example, where is it going to be? What is it going to do? And what's the purpose behind doing it? Be sure to ask your practitioner about any of the needles going in and about any of the moxa being burned; ideally you and your practitioner should be almost of one mind.

By changing some of the directions of acupuncture to accommodate certain patients' sensitivities, is it possible to still have a successful treatment?
As a CRPS patient, you should never feel as if someone is smarter and stronger about your condition than you are. If you have concerns about the location of needles or bodywork, you should always feel as if you are the captain of your ship in this regard.

You also perform what's called bodywork. What is this, and how does it complement acupuncture?
Bodywork is massage that simply helps the body to relax. It includes manipulating or holding the body with hands and lotion or instruments that help "get in" deeper, helping the body to feel what it's like to be relaxed and different. It's very helpful for folks with CRPS to realize what it is like to feel relaxed after so many months of stress and pain, and after all that's happened to them.

I've been trained as a massage practitioner, and this differs greatly from my training as an occupational therapist and as an acupuncturist. It's important that bodywork be done by someone who is qualified.

How can patients apply the principles of acupuncture within the practitioner's office to pain control outside in daily life?

I think there are a lot of things in Chinese medicine and Eastern philosophy's way of looking at nature that we can apply to our daily lives. We can drop the ruse that we are all the same, and what works for Betty has to work for all of us, just because it's the twenty-first century and we can have anything we want in an instant. The fact of the matter is, we are beings capable of pain, and oftentimes pain is a signal to us that we are wiser to listen rather than ignore. We are individuals who do better with support rather than trying to be isolated.

There are a lot of metaphors and realities in nature that we can look back at and realize there is a season for all things. It's inappropriate to go sledding in summertime, just as it's inappropriate for someone with CRPS in his hand to torture himself to learn piano. It's just not the season to do it. We can learn from Eastern medicine the perspective of time; that as we go on with our lives, there are cycles, there are seasons, there are things that change, and this moment that we are suffering through right now—this is not our whole life. Oftentimes we get caught up in thinking this is our whole life: this second, this suffering. Maybe not.

What else must CRPS patients do or change on their own in order to better manage themselves with CRPS—for however long it is in their lives?
I think two things are very important. One is that you again drop the misconception that anyone is smarter than you are, even if he or she has letters behind his or her name. You have to assert your own desires, your own worries, and you have to say what is important to you as a patient and not let people do things to you that you do not want to have done.

The second thing people need to do is be willing, open, and responsive to all types of things. You as a patient may be very surprised at what you find helps—and what doesn't help. It's important that you keep being open to trying amid all the grief and loss that accompanies CRPS. What may be helpful in the beginning of your recovery may not be helpful as your healing continues. I know it's difficult, but it's important to leave that door open.

Can any individual personality types address pain control and maintain balance in their lives differently? Do you have an example?
It's important to note that whatever works for your friend with CRPS—or someone online about whom you've read with CRPS—might not work for you. I think the amount of anxiety and fear and panic that can go into having CRPS can sometimes be overwhelming, and so breathing exercises, yoga, and movement exercises are often a way to move back into a feeling of calmness—a feeling of not going out of your mind.

If your patients could learn one thing from you about managing life with CRPS, what would it be?
It would be that your body is very wise, and that there is something it wants you to hear. You may not want to learn the lesson, and the lesson may be a very, very difficult lesson. It may be a lesson that literally turns your life upside down. That I have learned, and I have seen that our bodies are very wise.

Our bodies are sending us signals that we are wiser to listen to rather than just "kill." So, for example, I have a food allergy. While I hated it initially, it clearly has—every moment of every day—encouraged me to think about who I am and that I am a different kind of person. I'm not like everybody else. I've realized that and am true to that. It reminds me every moment of every day of the trueness of me, inside. I'm a wiser person because of it.

What do you think makes a good acupuncturist?
Amid all the different types of acupuncture, I think it's important to feel safe, trust that person, and be sure that person is qualified and knows what he's talking about. The acupuncturist should "speak" to you. He or she appreciates you, and you feel that.

I think what makes a good practitioner is knowing that the patients are really in charge, that they are going to leave the office doors and live their lives. It's not really up to the practitioner to become the Messiah or the curer or the greatest person on earth. It's important that the practitioner returns to you some things that you can do for yourself. The practitioner should always be looking toward the long term of what he or she can do to help the patient be more in control, feel better, and become wiser.

There are a lot of practitioners who may not fit you. Just keep looking. Again, I would just encourage you to keep hope alive and be willing to try new things and see who can be of help to you.

To be perfectly honest, a practitioner may not know much about CRPS; it's important that you educate them, and that you find out together what's most important. But again, it's important that you not think about yourself as a "CRPS case"—that you still think of yourself as the person you were born to be.

So the acupuncturist can simply work with the patient's description of CRPS, rather than being an expert in CRPS? He or she doesn't need to be an expert in the disease?
Yes. Don't think that this person is "out of it" if he or she has never heard of it before, but, true, you're going to want this person to read articles and do some research to find out how CRPS does affect you.

So he does not have to have treated CRPS before?
No, not necessarily.

What should patients who would like to try acupuncture for pain control do?
When evaluating a practitioner, you should be looking for a person who is understanding and whom you can trust. Try acupuncture on a limited basis—six to ten treatments, I think, are sufficient.

I think acupuncture is effective in pain control, but there is a whole bounty of benefits that acupuncture is probably better at producing than just pain control. Acupuncture is really much more about learning about yourself, about listening to yourself, not just having needles stuck in you. It's about becoming wise about who you are, rather than "Here's my arm; stick a needle in, and I will feel better." So go into it knowing that acupuncture has a whole bunch of other benefits beyond just easing the pain.

I hope these professionals have clarified some mysteries for you and offered an extended peek into how they view their healing crafts. Knowing each professional's strategy and treatment philosophy can better prepare you for the many bumps and turns on the CRPS road, as well as ensure that you trust your best interests in their hands. To learn more about your current doctor's and therapist's plans for you, try reading through the two chapters again, and see if you can predict how each of them would answer the questions posed in the interviews. Then, mark any unanswered questions and ask them at your next office visit.

It's important to remember that complementary therapies such as acupuncture can help by reducing troubling secondary symptoms like tension and anxiety. For more detailed information on this and other long-overlooked supportive treatments and services, let's go on to the next chapter, which focuses on complementary therapies.

A World of Support: Complementary Therapies

It may seem as if few people understand CRPS and that conventional medical options have not completely succeeded. Likewise, you may feel emotionally blindsided by pain and loss, and you may be baffled by how you're supposed to live with your diagnosis. Yet, although it's a little-known fact, a growing world of support is available to you. For pain relief, health sustenance, psychological strategies, and personal empowerment, you can turn to alternative sources to assist you in defending your life against CRPS's siege. In this chapter, you will learn about these sources so you don't have to stumble through the typical CRPS sufferer's long, tumultuous journey before discovering them.

Increasingly, traditional medicine is opening up to collaboration with complementary therapies, and numerous hospitals and medical schools now host alternative medicine across the nation. The term *alternative* has been changed to *complementary* or even *integrative* care in modern hospital settings, but whatever the terminology of the age, the rationale and benefits remain the same: treating the entire person rather than one specific part of the body. "Healing" involves physical, emotional, and psychological health, with various therapies focusing on more than one aspect of your well-being. There is a catch, however. Complementary therapies are not quick fixes, and they usually require your active participation as opposed to passive compliance.

Sufferers of CRPS require assistance on multiple fronts, with patients potentially benefiting greatly from adopting holistic methods that may assist the body in healing and regulating itself. Since conventional medicine has not yet produced a "cure" for CRPS, the addition of complementary therapy can be considered a valid and highly effective way to help the body heal and regulate itself. Like many prescribed pain medications and nerve membrane stabilizers, alternative options can ease discomfort and increase the chances for you to enter "remission." I, for example, feel that both acupuncture and Neurontin helped me tremendously, with each working differently on my pain.

Complementary medicine is not standardized and organized in the same manner as conventional medicine, so identifying options in your area and conferring with your doctor about treatments you would like to try outside his or her office becomes your responsibility. If your doctor is not familiar with one of the therapies described below, it does not mean that therapy is not a valid option. If you are interested in trying a certain therapy, work with your doctor to provide him or her with information about it so that you can assess together whether the treatment might work for your case. Easier said than done at times, of course, but if this effort fails, you can always seek the opinion of another specialist or contact the provider of the alternative therapy in your area. She or he can possibly help you in keeping your treatments integrated and—most important of all—ensure that all treatment providers remain in close communication. Some of the nation's most reputable pain-management clinics have already set the pace for this integrative model.

Occupational Therapy

While occupational therapy can often overlap with physical therapy, the philosophy behind this discipline involves more than just exercises or stretches; it also emphasizes the regaining of specific functions and achievement of goals that are personally meaningful to you. An occupational therapist can be a great guide in helping you relearn normal movements and sensations and can also provide specific, adaptive means for you to safely regain responsibility in your life. Maybe the therapist knows of a device that can help you hold a pen, a certain brace or "tent" to prevent your sheets from rubbing your leg at night, or any innovation for completing any task in an entirely different way from how you used to do it. An occupational therapist can gently help you work toward mobility and skin desensitization or teach you safe methods to slowly accomplish this on your own using materials such as towels, rice, or sponges.

Occupational therapists help you bridge the gap from disability to ability in a fast-paced, demanding world. While wondering how you can drive a car again, wash dishes differently, or maintain suppleness in your legs can prove overwhelming for you, your occupational therapist can devise inventive ways to work with your abilities and limitations and to get your life back—albeit a somewhat different life. Practitioners—whether they are generalists or specialists in such areas as neurology or hands—can be recommended by the organizations listed in the Resources section.

Bodywork/Massage

Bodywork and massage generally refer to various techniques of pressure, stroking, or other restorative activity applied to soft body tissue and muscle structure. Bodywork and massage practitioners can specialize in over two hundred specific techniques, such as Swedish massage and myofascial release (a gentle blend of stretching and massage). Bodywork can calm muscle spasms, release painful trigger points, help increase circulation, produce pain-buffering endorphins, and encourage normal brain circuitry and sensations. It is important, however, to notify the practitioner beforehand of your CRPS sensitivities and provide strict instructions on where to touch and not touch.

I was lucky enough to be treated by an occupational therapist who was also licensed in massage therapy and acupuncture, so treatment for all of my symptoms was well integrated by the same professional. I found slow myofascial release, petrissage (kneading, rolling, and picking up the skin and muscles), and effleurage (long, soothing, and stroking movements) helped me immensely with arm pain.

My desire to understand why and exactly how certain movements and massages helped relieve pain and increase pain endurance led to a very positive dialogue with my therapist. As I began healing and increasing activities, such as washing laundry and cooking, I noticed new aches and pains as my muscles formed and grew all over again; this was the stage at which massage was increasingly useful. Since my particular CRPS grew out of repetitive stress injuries in the upper extremities, I needed to ensure that I did not begin misusing my arms and hands as I'd done before. Since then, I've moved on to working with a medical massage therapist and a physical therapist familiar with manual therapy and trigger points. In all my work with these therapists, one fact is constant: Knowing your own muscles, off-limits areas, and pace is important in building a trusting relationship with these professionals.

Let's take a look at a few of the lesser-known forms of bodywork that other patients and I have found to be helpful.

Craniosacral Therapy

This is a gentle, hands-on treatment in which a therapist manipulates the soft tissue and bones of the head, the spine, and the pelvis; works with membranes that surround the bones; and clears blockages and corrects the flow of the cerebrospinal fluid. Practitioners assert that health problems develop when movement of the cerebrospinal fluid is blocked by trauma, strain, or dysfunctions in other parts of the body. Removal of these blockages can lead to reduced stress, improved sleep, increased energy, and enhanced organ function. To find a practitioner, check the Resources section.

Deborah found great relief through the use of gentle energy work such as craniosacral therapy. *Energy work* is a loosely applied term used to describe therapies that redirect and shape one's life energy to release obstructions, connect mind and body, enhance bodily system functioning, and enable the body to heal itself.

eborah's Story

My symptoms did not exactly match the usual definitions of CRPS. My problem did not start with a trauma, and I did not experience constant intense pain or pain in response to a puff of air. I did experience sufficient pain in my right foot when weight-bearing to put me in a wheelchair. My foot also changed color and temperature and was twitchy and hypersensitive. These feelings spread to my leg and my other foot.

My problem began in June of 2002. After various, conflicting doctors' opinions, I was diagnosed with RSD in October. I began physical therapy with a therapist who was trained in acupuncture and tai chi. I also began going to a person who practiced craniosacral therapy and other "energy work." I also had a sympathetic block, which did not help, and started taking nortriptyline, which did.

I have gone from being unable to walk without crutches in October 2002 to being able to do all my daily tasks now, including walking a mile or so at a time, although I have some mild symptoms that continue to diminish.

I am convinced that the energy work, with which I had no experience before this crisis, was vital in my improvement.

Zero-Balancing

Focusing on the mind-body relationship between energy and the body's physical structures, this type of bodywork is a newer practice that was developed in 1973 by an osteopath named Fritz Smith. It is a gentle, hands-on practice in which the therapist progressively evaluates and balances the skeletal structure, joints, and soft tissues. Balancing is conducted side-to-side on the shoulders, scapulae, back muscles, and all the way down to the hips and feet. Pressure may be placed on spasms, causing imbalances on one side or the other, until ultimately a more whole, integrated state resides in the patient. Information on finding a practitioner can be found in the Resources section of this book.

Trigger Point Therapy

With repetitive stress injuries, as with many types of aches and pains, discomfort can often be traced back to trigger points. These points form as tiny knots in the fascia of muscles, oftentimes placing pressure on nerves and potentially causing pain at the knot site and along the nerve. As a result, trigger points, when activated, can cause referred pain patterns. In other words, the pain may emerge somewhere other than the site of the trigger point, which is why medical professionals are often perplexed as to why you have pain in your wrist if the trigger points are in your forearm. The recommended trigger point therapy method for a CRPS patient is very gentle: A physical therapist or skilled medical massage therapist applies pressure or gently massages the painful spots, with the eventual goal of applying ischemic pressure and deactivating the spots over time. This method, also called myotherapy, is also effective in managing fibromyalgia. An excellent book that demystifies myofascial pain and dysfunction is *The Trigger Point Therapy Workbook: Your Self-Treatment Guide for Pain Relief* by Clair Davies. It is the recently released patient version of Travell and Simons's heavyweight medical reference, *Myofascial Pain and Dysfunction: The Trigger Point Manual*.

I can share that once my burning pain was under control, trigger point therapy brought me back to life over the past few years and helps keeps me functioning. My muscles tend to have difficulty letting go of a spasm, which, unchecked, can easily snowball into nerve and fascial sensations to create a pain cycle.

Manual Lymphatic Drainage (MLD) Therapy

Originating in Europe in the 1930s, lymphatic drainage therapy can help manage edema, or swelling. An MLD-certified massage therapist gently and slowly massages a patient's superficial fascia to create a pumping action in the lymphatic vessels. This flushes out the stagnant lymphatic fluid and reduces pain, enabling more movement in the area. The therapist can also pump the lymph farther away from the affected area if direct touch to that area is intolerable.

Acupuncture

Acupuncture, as discussed in the previous chapter, involves the rechanneling of your energy to restore balance and calm to your mind, body, and spirit. It releases pain-fighting beta-endorphins. If you are squeamish about needles or do not believe in the procedure's effectiveness, I still urge you to try it. Over time, your body will become more receptive to the effects of acupuncture, with some effects taking place immediately after a treatment and others needing more time to sink in. As someone who used to pass out at the mere sight of a needle, I recall my first acupuncture visit, at which I asked, sniffling with anticipation and desperation, "Do I have to believe in acupuncture for it to work?" The answer was a resounding, "No." Regardless of what I originally thought or believed, the acupuncture created pain relief without me having to adopt a new philosophy.

Acupuncture's effects extend to the emotional body as well. While each acupuncturist's style is different, acupuncture can transform frustration, anxiety, and panic into a peacefulness that can withstand the contagious energy of fear. This does not mean that your acupuncturist becomes a psychologist or that acupuncture requires talk therapy to be effective; however, in explaining what type of pain you're experiencing, you will find your emotions and perceptions are intimately tied to your physical descriptions.

Acupuncture greatly facilitated my healing and continues to provide potent, holistic relief for my case. When I step off the treatment table and exit a session of acupuncture, I sense I've passed through an enormously condensed exorcism of pain, as well as the anxiety and grief that go with it. On my worst days, when the horrible electrical sensations were revving through my arms at a roar, a back treatment could quiet them to the point at which my mind could take over and push them into the background. An enormous weight would be lifted from my interior spirit and mood, leaving my whole being floating on nothing but peacefulness and calm. Following a treatment, the choked sob constantly lurking at the back of my throat, the tightness in my chest, and the constant struggle to block out the endless questions I have about my condition are cleansed and purged. My inner calm is restored and remains untouched by any brain chatter, shallow breathing, stomach upset, or muscle tightness that so quickly tumbles into and torments my "core" on any given day.

If I *try* to worry or focus on a painful area—just to test the extent of acupuncture's effects—I find its effects are indeed stronger than my efforts. Finally, it requires more energy to induce worry and pain than it does to resist it. I feel then as if anything is possible again; nothing can touch my peacefulness and harmony, nurtured and guarded by this treatment. My spirit can soar again.

Please remember that the efficacy of different treatments can also depend on what was the initial noxious event or underlying injury that led you to CRPS. For me, I had coexisting median and ulnar nerve problems due to repetitive stress injuries from typing (and careless physical therapy). Many repetitive stress injuries, such as carpal tunnel syndrome, respond well to acupuncture. For more insights on acupuncture, read the interview with Sheri Barnes (Chapter 5). To find a licensed acupuncturist, check the Resources section.

TENS Unit

The transdermal electrical nerve stimulation, or TENS, unit is a small, portable box with electrodes that you attach to or near painful areas of your body. The box emits intermittent electrical currents through the electrodes, interfering with pain messages and potentially "resetting" your affected nerves to make them fire less frequently. Use of the TENS unit can also reduce muscle spasms around sore areas, thereby reducing the chances that chain reactions of spasms will occur.

Ask if you can borrow, rent, or buy a TENS unit from your doctor and then experiment with the level of stimulation to find the most pain relief. If at first you don't feel as if you are succeeding, try placing the electrodes elsewhere, at a lower degree, or at a different modulation. At times, I find the tingling sensation caused by the currents just distract me from the pain, while at other times—especially on rainy days—it just adds extra, painful stimulation. Some say that replacing your perception of pain with the perception of tingling is beneficial in itself, because doing so interrupts repetitive pain messages to the brain. So, I use the unit in relation to what will work on a particular day.

Biofeedback

Biofeedback is a treatment and re-education system that enables you to monitor your own biological and physiological state and learn how to control it in many respects. With the help of a specialist, patients learn how to relax, increase the temperature of a limb, reduce heart rate, and evaluate the body's chronic overactivity or hyperarousal so that it can be reduced or returned to normal. Pain, mood, and sleeping patterns can be regulated through trained concentration. During training, patients learn to monitor their biofeedback signals via body sensors and electrodes that are hooked up to a biofeedback machine.

This new awareness of otherwise habitual symptoms and states can help patients reduce troublesome physical symptoms. Patients can use their relaxation tools at home, remembering to see their emotions as a choice rather than as an automatic reaction to their physical symptoms. Dr. Donna Gillette, director of the Stress and Pain Management Clinic of North Florida and a CRPS patient herself, says biofeedback is a "technique for how to be 'in touch' with your body—without being consumed by it."

Brenda, whose story appears in Chapter 1, shares the following details about her experience with biofeedback:

> About five months after I felt the first symptoms of CRPS, I began learning biofeedback and the process of raising my body temperature in one area. Biofeedback is only effective if my pain level is at a five or less (on a scale of one to ten). Using biofeedback, I can reduce or push back a migraine, I can raise the temperature in my legs ten-plus degrees, and I can have twenty minutes twice a day that are peaceful and pain-free. Achieving these results took six months to learn. Biofeedback does take time, daily, to practice, and it was best having someone who understands pain teach it to me. I think you can shape biofeedback to fit your belief system, as I did. I made the process into more of a combination of meditating on scripture verses and praise.

You'll find many types of feedback, depending on the particular physiological system being targeted. For example, EMG muscle biofeedback focuses on controlling muscular contractions, thermal biofeedback focuses on controlling the temperature of an extremity, and electroencephalograph (EEG) biofeedback, or neurofeedback, focuses on the central nervous system's activity.

Doctors using biofeedback with their CRPS patients claim that roughly 15 to 60 percent of their patients have found effective pain relief using this drug-free, noninvasive practice. It's important to note, as Brenda points out, that biofeedback takes a significant time to learn for it to be effective. Many pain-management centers and private practices use biofeedback. If your doctor does not use this technique, you can ask for a prescription to seek it elsewhere.

Meditation

Meditation places pain reduction within your control because the only tool you need to carry out this treatment is your own mind. A perfect example of mind-body-spirit relatedness, meditation actually reduces the stress hormone cortisol, lowers heart rate, and increases production of melatonin and serotonin, both known for their calming qualities. As an added benefit, the altered consciousness of meditation enables you to observe and manage your fears and anger with secure detachment.

Although the idea of meditating might initially put you off, you do not have to be a Buddhist, new-age enthusiast, or introspective type to try this technique. Anyone with CRPS has had to look deeply inside, so if you're reading this book, you are probably ready to try some form of meditation. It's also something that you can do for yourself—and it doesn't cost anything.

Getting Started

Meditation has many different methods and approaches, with wide room for you to customize what works for you. You can focus on breathing, visualization, repetition of certain affirmative phrases or sounds, or progressive relaxation. People have their own preferred perceptive pathways; that is, they may be more visual, auditory, or even tactile. You can use your personal preference in choosing your form of meditation.

Here's a simple way to get started on a meditation practice. Keep a guided meditation or relaxing, wordless song on your phone or media device, or a book on your bedside with some passages for meditation that you like. Play the song—either a meditation journey or music—or read a few pages from the book. Now close your eyes, lie back, and focus on the gift of mind/soul expansion that your brief respite and distance will give you. Know that you don't need to "believe" in it for it to have an impact on your brain. Your mind may drift, and you may fall asleep for a moment. You may find that your own meditations develop and help you better than guided ones. Try more than one method and don't abandon the practice until you have actively tried it for a while. You can do it for a few minutes to recenter yourself, or engage in a half hour of practice when the pain surges.

To encourage your meditation practice, try setting aside one spot in your home that you find beautiful and calming. Make this place your sanctuary, and associate it only with positive, creative, nurturing symbols. When I was recuperating in Baltimore, I used to sit in front of a large window that looked out onto its harbor. The light of the moon and its reflection on the water provided a magnificent view that I found quieting and almost spiritual in its grace. Now I meditate in my den, seated on a calming green Persian carpet and surrounded by books that I love. For more ideas on enhancing your chosen space, check Chapter 7, "Dynamite Distractions."

The practice of mindfulness meditation has become increasingly common as a technique for managing both stress and pain, and accessible resources now abound on this topic. I have listed some meditation resources in the Resources section at the back of this book.

Breathing and the Relaxation Response

Ever notice how shallow your breathing becomes when you're panicked? Deep breathing promises relaxation, and a simple breathing exercise used by mind-body treatment experts has been found to reduce the stressful fight-or-flight response revving in your nervous system. Called the "relaxation response," and coined by Herbert Benson of the Mind-Body Medical Institute, it is achieved by a specific breathing pattern that causes physiological changes, nervous system relaxation, and a winding down of sympathetic activity. While it can bring an immediate sense of calm to you, the long-term benefits are the most valuable and are attainable by performing a simple exercise for twenty minutes, two times a day, for several weeks. Use the following procedure:

1. Find a quiet environment and sit or lie down comfortably.

2. Start by thinking of nothing but how it feels for the air to move into and out of your nostrils as you breathe. Breathe into your stomach rather than your chest. Place your hands on your stomach and feel how it rises and falls with the movement of air.

3. Once your breathing is deep and steady and your body is relaxed, focus for ten to twenty minutes on a simple mental device, such as the word *one* or a brief prayer.

4. During the exercise, assume a passive attitude toward intrusive thoughts. That is, don't hang on to them, but don't try to force them out of your mind, either. Simply notice any thoughts as they arise and then allow them to float away, as though you were watching them drift down a river and out of your field of vision.

(Adapted from *Beyond the Relaxation Response,* Herbert Benson, MD.)

Affirmative Statements and Mantras

I have created certain affirmations to remind myself that I'm a separate entity from my pain. Try these affirmations a few times, and if they don't resonate deeply with you, see if you can devise adaptations that have more personal meaning, such as a short prayer from childhood or a line from a favorite song.

Affirmation 1:

I am larger than my pain.
My emotions extend deeper and wider than my pain.
My mind can explore entire worlds beyond my pain.

My spirit is grander and higher than my pain.
(Repeat ten times.)

Sometimes, when I felt I was losing my entire personality to pain, I'd simply remind myself of the inner "Elena":

Affirmation 2:
My personality can shine through pain's walls.
(Repeat ten or more times.)

Finally, another affirmative meditation you can try before bedtime is the following:

Affirmation 3:
Pain is not me, and I am not pain.
I can think higher,
see lower,
and dream beyond my pain.
(Repeat ten times.)

Modifications

Perhaps thinking of pain and drawing attention to yourself can incite anxiety and unease rather than relief. As an alternative, try thinking of an external, soothing image, such as a fresh flower, a soft kitten, or how it feels to hug a special loved one. Imagine you're breathing in a comforting, delicious aroma and focus on how that makes you feel. If you choose a pleasant, calming image or memory to focus on, it's best to ensure that this image does not represent something that has been affected by the onset of your CRPS experience. I found focusing on trips or certain relationships too upsetting, because they touched worries that these people and experiences were out of my grasp due to CRPS. Instead, I chose a childhood memory from camp, which represented a very happy, secure time in my life and was somewhat immune to CRPS's effects.

Experiment, and keep trying. See what tricks work for you to start sensing a detachment from your current situation and explore this state of calm. Make meditation a habit every day and give it time!

Meditation and Faith

In Herbert Benson's *Beyond the Relaxation Response* he asserts that adding faith to traditional relaxation-response breathing exercises greatly enhances its benefits for patients. Indeed, turning to your religion can significantly enlarge your circle of community support, guidance, and personal sense of strength. For many of us, however, adding the ingredient of belief is easier said than done. Since claiming a solid, static faith is not a simple feat for many of us, perhaps a new slant on the concept of faith can help you over this bump in the road and expand your approach to introspective relaxation.

Have you ever imagined that faith can be considered a process rather than a possession? At times, you may sense flickers of divinity or connectivity in your midst, but at other times, faith seems far away. Maybe you *feel* a reassuring sense of connectivity to something greater than yourself at times, but it disappears as soon as you try to stare at in the face and *analyze* it. Perhaps you attend a religious service, and while you feel better in the environment of beauty and goodwill it conveys, you disagree with the words in your prayer book. How can you resolve this conflict to your healthful benefit?

Rather than intellectually attempting to correlate these conflicting sides of yourself, seek out those moments of feeling and accept them—in whatever form or combination they take. In times of heartbreak and suffering, your need to find strength and solace can also be transformed into a gift of unprecedented receptivity. Maybe it's time to try another congregation or just construct your own personal practice of nurturing this hope to fill your heart.

Personally, this has been a struggle to which I've only recently found a solution amid my trials with CRPS. I have accepted that I am a woman of erratic faith. Yet, I have stopped trying to create a master sense of everything as it relates to my belief system and have simply accepted the prayers, inspiring words, environment, songs, and ethics that fill my heart. I recognize that I need this extra strength more than I need to rationalize why I receive it. Similarly, while you might have the right to be angry or frustrated about your condition, the practice of remaining calm is more important because your body needs the tranquility. In the case of chronic illness, the ends (faith, strength, solace, encouragement) justify the means (religion, belief system, music, poetry) every single day. And each day is a new day to start over again.

Part of recognizing faith as a process includes being open to accepting new sources of hope when the old ones stop offering significant meaning. Rather than worrying about your belief systems failing, remember how many sources have yet to be discovered. Just as certain treatments are not considered ineffective simply because they do not benefit you every time, so too may different sources of hope click on and off with you, depending on your needs and phases of life. Experiment and keep yourself open to what feels right—if even for just a day or a season. You can always circle back or hone your own new hybrid system of beliefs.

Hypnotherapy

Ancient Chinese and Egyptians used hypnosis in religious rituals and to encourage healing. Now, leading pain-management centers, such as Johns Hopkins Hospital, include hypnotherapy as a valid, effective treatment for pain management, and the National Institutes of Health has just launched a trial to evaluate the effectiveness of hypnosis in pain management. Combining deep relaxation of the conscious mind with focused concentration, hypnotherapy works on the subconscious while the conscious mind remains passive. In this state, suggestions can be made to your subconscious in order to reprogram basic behaviors, attitudes, and perceptions according to your personal or more desirable ideals (e.g., perception of pain reduction). As a result, your conscious mind accepts these ideals as reality.

Hypnosis unfortunately carried the stigma of magic shows and artificiality for many years, but it's important to remember that daydreaming and meditating also present states of altered consciousness. Remain open to all the options your mind offers you in managing CRPS. For more information on finding a hypnotherapist or practicing it on your own, check the Resources section.

Yoga

Rather than an esoteric practice reserved only for those who can put their feet behind their heads, yoga is "meditation in motion" and is available to everyone. Like meditation, yoga can still the mind, calm the nervous system, and enhance defenses against pain. However, sometimes it is easier to relax by focusing on the gentlest and slowest of movements rather than by sitting and focusing during pure meditation.

While pain and life stresses associated with CRPS deplete your sense of "wholeness" and equilibrium, yoga positions, or *asanas*, provide physical, mental, and spiritual rejuvenation and create a sense of calm unity. Just as hormones can affect your emotions or anxiety can cause a tightened chest or headache, yoga can fortify all aspects of your self. According to Yogacharya Iyengar, a leading international authority on hatha yoga, "Yogic science believes the nerves control the unconscious mind and that when the nervous system is strong, a person faces stressful situations more positively. Asanas improve blood flow to all the cells of the body and revitalize the nerve cells. This flow strengthens the nervous system and its capacity for enduring stress." Through its combination of postures and breathing practices, called *pranayama*, yoga can also gradually increase your strength, muscle control, and flexibility.

Yoga follows the principal that there is untapped divinity within each of us, offering a secular means for everyone to embrace spirituality. Much like other faiths, it can open a door for you to release your attachment to negative thoughts and emotions and fill yourself with peace, security, and hope. This can once again equip you with better defenses against pain and its related thoughts and emotions, breaking the cycle in which pain and anxiety feed off one another.

Many types of yoga exist, though the Western interest in yoga has focused primarily on the various practices of hatha yoga, such as Kripalu. Remember, even two or three movements while seated in a chair constitute yoga postures if done consciously. For the gentlest of movements, look for a restorative or Kripalu yoga class. To try a yoga session, contact your local yoga center, fitness club, or hospital to inquire about classes that accommodate people with chronic pain. You'll know if your teacher is the right one for you by your intuition; request that she or he offer modifications for your specific limitations.

Finally, if getting to the yoga class provides more stress than you need, use a video at home and pace yourself regularly—or try it when you feel a flare-up coming on. For months, I could bear to complete only two movements shown in a seated yoga video; after nine months, I was performing eleven! It takes time. Check the Resources section of this book for several gentle yoga videos and books.

Qigong

Qigong (pronounced "chee gung") is an ancient Chinese practice that combines movement, meditation, breathing, and visualization for mind-body-spirit wellness. You can practice these simple, vital energy movements easily at home by following a video or book (try *Qigong for Living* by Yanling Lee Johnson) or by working with a practitioner. See the Resources section for more information.

Tai Chi

This is a form of meditation that uses healing movement to circulate chi (energy). Tai chi features slow, fluid movements and breathing that can be made with muscle control, fluidity, and balance. You can try an online video at home or attend a class at your health club or hospital. Tai chi is increasingly offered as a beneficial and gentle therapy for many medical conditions.

Feldenkrais Method

Often used for patients with multiple sclerosis and cerebral palsy, the Feldenkrais Method is a movement therapy that can help restore normal movement without strain. Its aim is to encourage new awareness of one's neuromuscular patterns and rigidities that may have become habitual due to pain-avoidant behavior and protective positioning of an area sensitive to touch. Feldenkrais is a very gentle practice, available in two forms: group classes, called "awareness through movement," and individual therapy, called "functional integration." In functional integration, the practitioner works in a hands-on fashion, helping you harness the power of your central nervous system and explore comfort in movement and touch again. Websites for finding a practitioner are listed in the Resources section.

Light Therapy

Light therapies use infrared light to penetrate trigger points, painful areas, or the spinal cord, encouraging circulation and nerve function to engender healing. According to Dr. Connie Haber, a CRPS laser therapist and original researcher of the FDA-approved microlight, "Light travels along the neural axis and improves communication between the sympathetic and parasympathetic nervous systems. Once they start speaking to one another again, the patient finds relief." Treatments normally last ten minutes and bypass the risks associated with lasers by functioning on the same principles as low-level laser devices.

Professionals trained in laser therapy claim a 65 to 90 percent success rate in providing relief and improvement in CRPS patients. However, like every other CRPS treatment, laser therapy is not guaranteed to work for everyone. Patients who have had a sympathectomy face particular challenges, and roughly 10 to 20 percent of these patients can find their CRPS exacerbated by the treatments. To test its effectiveness, Haber recommends trying three treatments; if you do not find improvement, you should stop.

The FDA has approved several light-therapy devices that are used to treat ailments ranging from carpal tunnel syndrome to torn ligaments. These devices include the Photonic Stimulator and the Anodyne laser. As light therapy becomes more common in the treatment of chronic pain, arthritis, and soft-tissue injuries, North American medical professionals are showing a growing interest in learning about it and including it in their practices. The U.S. Olympic track and field team has used light therapy to treat its athletes. Check in the Resources section to find a provider.

Hyperbaric Oxygen

Hyperbaric oxygen (HBO) therapy operates on the principle of increasing oxygen levels to saturate the blood and water in the body in order to recharge the body with oxygen. In daily life, we breathe air that is 21 percent oxygen. Face masks can provide 100 percent oxygen, while a pressurized chamber of pure oxygen can provide two to three times this amount of naturally occurring oxygen. The result is up to fifteen more times more oxygen flow to injured tissues and assistance in the preservation of damaged tissue. White blood cells' ability to kill bacteria is enhanced, thereby reducing local swelling and promoting the growth of new blood vessels.

During treatment, which is painless and lasts roughly one hour, patients enter a hyperbaric chamber that provides conditions for breathing oxygen equivalent to thirty-three feet underwater. Patients can read, listen to music, or just rest—and they might feel a bit of pressure in their ears, similar to the sensation of being in an airplane. The patient remains in the chamber while his or her oxygen levels go up from 80 to 100 mmHg (millimeters of mercury) to 1,800 to 2,000 mmHg.

Hyperbaric oxygen treatments are available at many hospitals and are normally used with burn victims, patients with multiple sclerosis, osteoporosis, infections, and a few other limited conditions such as decompression sickness and air embolisms. In the United Kingdom, the Multiple Sclerosis Society has opened its hyperbaric oxygen treatments center doors specifically to CRPS patients. Hyperbaric oxygen may not help with every CRPS case, but its benefits are noted for symptoms such as swelling. For more information, check the Resources section.

Natural Creams, Oils, and Soaks

Topical, natural therapeutics are highly accessible options to consider, even if just for a supportive, tingling distraction or an add-on to an existing regimen. They may or may not work miracles, but being able to reduce your pain level by one or two notches is significant when every bit counts.

Epsom Salts

Epsom salts work naturally as calcium channel blockers to reduce pain. Use two cups of the salts for an entire bath or soak painful areas in a sink or basin containing one half to one cup of the salts for up to twenty minutes. Epsom salts are available in any drugstore.

Nonprescription Gels

Sombra gel combines natural plant extracts, such as green tea extract and grapefruit seed extract with menthol, camphor, and capsaicin, to relieve inflammation, distract patients from muscle pain, and help joint soreness. Massage the gel directly onto the affected areas. It is available only through health professionals, but you can go to www.sombrausa.com to inquire about ordering its retail equivalent.

Arnica is a flower that can be infused in massage oil or added to a cream. *Arnica montana* is also available as a homeopathic supplement (pills) and is effective for injuries. It is available at most health-food stores.

Finally, Biofreeze contains an herbal extract from a South American holly shrub and can aid muscular discomfort, replacing pain with a cold, tingling sensation. I find that putting Biofreeze on my neck can help even with muscular spasm–induced headaches. Visit www.biofreeze.com for information on ordering and ask your physical therapist for free samples.

Psychological Counseling

Whether you are locked in a minute-by-minute struggle with the pain and finding the courage to go on or you are gnawed to your core by the uncertainties of your physical, financial, and social state, every person with CRPS needs some psychosocial support to get through this roller coaster time. New ways of looking at your life, reframing losses, developing coping mechanisms for specific challenges and setbacks, and cultivating a new form of self-esteem are invaluable tools for healing. Both individual and group therapy sessions can remind you that you're not alone, your feelings and thoughts are normal for your situation, and you can learn to manage yourself.

Depression and Pain

The experience of pain goes deeper than just skin and bones. It carries numerous emotional associations and fears with it. It causes heartbreak, grief, intense anxiety, and depression. In an article from the *Journal of Clinical Psychiatry* Dr. Nelson Hendler says, "Chronic pain almost always leads to depression: This is normal." Likewise, despite the tendency of some doctors to dismiss pain as being psychogenic when surgery or treatment does not bring desired results, Hendler writes, "Depression is rarely manifested by chronic pain."

Hendler describes four stages of a patient's psyche through his or her struggle with chronic pain:

0–2 months: This is the acute stage in which the patient expects an injury to pass, and she or he is not clinically depressed.

2–6 months: The subacute stage is when panic sets in. "Why is this happening? Why am I not getting better?" The patient begins extensive questioning about his or her treatment and diagnosis, which is a legitimate response to unrelenting pain.

6 months–8 years: This is the chronic stage. With the comprehension that the pain may be permanent, the patient becomes markedly depressed.

3–12 years: The subchronic stage features adaptive strategies and functional adjustments to managing a life in which pain may persist, regardless of whether the patient is pleased with his lot or not. Depression is significantly reduced or completely gone.

Working Through Difficult Issues

Losing normal function in a limb and the possibility of having to use a walker or wheelchair can wreak havoc on your self-image, sense of attractiveness, and sense of power. A counselor can help you work through this pain and reshape the foundations of some basic conceptions of self that can help ease this transition. A counselor can also help you tackle pain-related fear. This is particularly important because fear of further injury or re-injury can lead to the guarding of an affected area, which in turn can compound functional challenges.

Grief over your life as it was, your previous ease of function, your old self, a job you loved, the change in your relationships, and the loss of your dreams are also matters that your therapist can help you wade through. While it is important to maintain a positive attitude, you must also allow yourself to recognize and validate your grief. Even after you've passed through the eye of the storm, you may need long-term help pushing through your grief.

A counselor can also help you work with anger. I remember being angry not only at the health professionals who had over-looked my condition and the workers' compensation insurance that complicated my life, but also at my own caregivers. I felt like a caged bird, and I was a match that could flare at any provocation. This, in turn, caused horrible feelings of guilt over not handling my situation more gracefully.

Little did I know, CRPS is something we manage the best we can—and everyone falls from grace from time to time. As you move back into your life, possibly altered, counseling may help you through other emotional and psychological trauma you may carry from the experience.

Getting Started

Imagine the complications in the mix when a CRPS patient has initially been accused of suffering psychogenic or psychosomatic pain. Would the stigma of that initial insult keep you from seeking psychological help later on in your struggle?

Counselors can be invaluable in helping you set realistic goals for yourself and preventing catastrophic thinking whenever you falter in this journey. Short-term crisis counseling and cognitive-behavioral counseling can be especially helpful in devising ways for you to reevaluate challenges you come across and how you act and think in response to them. Do you think in black-and-white terms about your life and your setbacks with CRPS? It takes effort and conscious guidance to train yourself to avoid resorting to declarations that you "cannot do anything," "will never see a better day," "will never be loved," "will never work again," "are completely ruined," and other automatic thoughts that can hold you back.

For more information on psychologists and counselors, contact some of the organizations listed in the Resources section. A wonderful workbook for examining your thought processes and working to reframe them is *Managing Pain Before It Manages You* by Margaret Caudill.

Art Therapy

Pain provides its own hyperactive, frantically negative form of mind-body-spirit energy. If you harness this energy to fuel creative expression, the pleasure of unleashing it and creating something new can offer your heart and soul a sense of liberation and boundlessness.

Oftentimes artistic expression is the only way that some patients can present how a pain feels, both physically and emotionally. Art, like prayer, comes from the same source: the heart. Many people, such as Dr. Erv Hinds in *A Life Beyond Pain,* would dare say the heart is synonymous with the soul. Using this interpretation, art therapy—either under the guidance of a trained art therapist or on your own—can aid you immensely in this journey.

Maybe it's working with a color that brings you peace or symbolizes relief, or perhaps you wish to draw how you have come to feel or see yourself—positively or negatively. Instead of tracking your pain verbally in a journal, you may prefer to document your feelings in drawings. Make an art and healing journal, with no expectations of doing anything but being true to yourself. An advanced therapeutic exercise in making peace with where you are could be creating a collage that mixes images of things you've lost with things you have gained during your dealings with CRPS.

These ideas and others are available for you to explore. For more information, see Chapter 7 "Dynamite Distractions" or the Resources section.

Writing

At the risk of repeating myself on the topic of the importance of writing, using prose and poetry to express your feelings can also help you work through difficult times. Writing can provide you with a way to personally construct meaning and order amidst all the chaos and uncertainty that you feel in your life due to CRPS. As a result of both my own experience and those of patients who have written to me with their stories, writing about fears helps to break them down. This is not to say that this practice will eliminate them, but, rather, that it will help you look them in the face and then control them in the abstract. By recording fears, I purge myself of the energy it takes to actively entertain them—at least for the day. I can shrug my shoulders at them with a bit of detachment. Suggestions for keeping a pain journal are included in Chapter 3.

Naturopathic and Homeopathic Medicine

The practice of using natural medications and herbs has been around for centuries. Naturopathic medicine uses a holistic approach to enable a person to take charge of his or her own healing; naturopathic doctors incorporate homeopathy, diet and lifestyle changes, bodywork, preventive education, and other methods to encourage the body's innate ability to heal itself. Meanwhile, homeopathy follows the principle of strengthening the body through consumption of very diluted solutions of the same substances that at full strength would cause disease symptoms in a healthy person.

Unfortunately few allopathic doctors know which herbs or natural medications could interact with powerful prescription drugs; likewise, homeopathic and naturopathic practitioners are not always sufficiently knowledgeable of all potential interactions. If you have utilized medications for quite some time and wish to support your body with more natural remedies, take your time in learning about them; natural or prescription, the substances are potent, and should not be purchased or taken without the advice of a physician.

Consult with a practitioner who will work with you to learn about your condition, examine your particular medications, and customize a plan for your optimal health. Sources for learning more and for finding a practitioner are available in the Resources section.

Moving Forward: Rehabilitation Services and Disability Employment

Many states have their own department of rehabilitation services, an undiscovered resource for many people trying to regain their independence. It may take a while to obtain a first appointment, but rehabilitation services provide you with no-cost access to an unbiased group of professionals whose sole aim is to help you function as optimally and as easily as possible. From occupational therapy to technology assistance and workforce support, they provide problem-solving strategies to each patient and dedicate an unbelievable amount of time toward meeting specific needs. State rehab officers can brainstorm new careers for you, alert you to part-time or work-from-home partnerships, and provide you with training in the use of new assistive technologies or in skills needed for certain careers. They can also work with your lawyer or workers' compensation caseworker to coordinate the transition back into the workforce.

While I was lucky enough to benefit from Maryland's highly comprehensive program, many other states have comparable programs or solicit private agencies to fulfill your needs. If you have a workers' compensation case, try—if possible—to use your state rehabilitation program instead of workers' compensation. The state program will have only your best interests at heart and can provide more suggestions for returning to the workplace than most private insurance company vocational rehab programs allow. Also, state rehabilitation services can specifically assist with job place-ment via their own resources or outsourced consultants; this "job placement" service often does not fall within the parameters of "vocational rehabilitation" under workers' compensation. Check the small print of your state's workers' compensation policy to en-sure (and to prove to your state rehab department) that you are not entitled to job placement assistance via worker's compensation.

As you move forward, I suggest that you resist the urge to settle your workers' compensation case early, until you know that you will be able to obtain health insurance coverage elsewhere for your condition. Closing your case—depending on the state—leaves you at high risk for unpredictable, ongoing medical costs that could be dismissed as a "pre-existing condition" under other insurance policies. I opted to waive weekly compensation while I eased back into the job market in a less hand-intensive career direction, test-ing my endurance while knowing my medical care would remain completely covered until my condition stabilized. Hopefully, once full health coverage truly becomes a stable cornerstone of Ameri-can society, this problem will become a relic of the past in the United States.

If you're stepping out on your own in the job search, the Social Security Administration sponsors a disability employment service that offers a wealth of information on your rights as a potential em-ployee, where to look for leads, and how to go about finding proper employment. You can also have your disability rating evaluated by a state vocational office, which actually can provide you with an advantage in applying for a government job (appointed rather than competitive position), even if you were rejected for Social Security disability benefits. If you can work with adaptive aids and relatively consistent work modifications, this is something to con-sider. Check out http://choosework.net/about and www.opm.gov /policy-data-oversight/disability-employment.

I'd like to end this discussion of complementary treatments with stories from two patients whose experiences illustrate how mixing several different conventional and complementary therapies can be beneficial—indeed, crucial—in successfully managing CRPS/RSD. In Tracy's story, take note of how many different and varied treatment methods she has utilized: acupuncture, psychotherapy, pharmaceuticals, nerve blocks, and Epsom salts, among others. Jill's story illustrates the dramatic strides one can make in improvement, even after having been wheelchair-bound. It also emphasizes the importance of trying many different therapies and personal coping strategies until you hit on the right combination for your particular case.

racy's Story

Five years ago I was in a car accident. The airbag crushed against my left hand and lower right jaw. My life was forever changed from that moment in time. I was fortunate because the orthopedic surgeon who treated me soon realized that the physical therapy I was receiving in his office was not specialized enough for my condition. He encouraged me to see a hand surgeon and to start therapy with a certified hand therapist and continue with a physical therapist as well. At the time, he tried to explain what CRPS was and what type of treatments I might need to pursue.

I am thankful for my early diagnosis. The hand surgeon recommended acupuncture, Nikken magnets, and grape seed extract for my immune system. The magnets drained my energy field in a negative way, but the acupuncture had some benefit. Acupuncture helped with the tremendous swelling and discoloration in addition to increasing the circulation. Being hypersensitive due to the CRPS made acupuncture rather uncomfortable for me; they had to put in a lot of needles in a variety of areas that were sensitive and very swollen. I felt like a porcupine, but I proceeded and am glad I did. It was recommended that I get treatment two to three times a week for four to six weeks.

During that time, I started to see a physiatrist (a doctor who specializes in physical rehabilitation) on a regular basis who helped me decipher the different treatments and medicines. This doctor became the catalyst that helped lead me onto the path of wellness.

After trial and error with interscalene nerve blocks, which for me were lifesavers, I was encouraged to find a psychotherapist who could help me learn to cope with the permanency of the CRPS. My physiatrist and my anesthesiologist both recommended this course to me. So I found a psychotherapist who was also a medical family therapist. RSD had taken me on a roller-coaster ride of emotions. It isolated me socially and sent me into recurring bouts of depression. She taught me, through hypnotherapy, to develop stress-management and relaxation techniques that I am still using today, five years later.

I underwent numerous trigger point injections over the next few years; they helped ease some of the complications from spasms. And I was constantly looking and trying other alternative therapies along the way. Some of them led to success, while others fizzled out over time. CRPS is like a long, winding roller coaster [ride], and we should never stop looking for successful treatments!

Over these last five years, I have been on a variety of different medicines. At this time, I use Neurontin daily. When necessary, I use Valium, Mobic, Lidoderm patches, and speed gel (a custom anti-inflammatory topical). Having CRPS has taught me to always proceed with caution, to limit myself, and to try to understand what my body is capable of. At first I was always looking for a quick fix. So my doctors and therapists encouraged me to experiment with a variety of treatments and therapies and decide what was beneficial to me.

I find warm Epsom-salt baths soothing, so I even take these to loosen up before I go to some therapies. I was a very active person before I had CRPS, and I had been taking some yoga classes as well. I wanted to be able to increase my levels of activity when the vicious cycle of pain would allow me to do so. So I found a restorative yoga class. This practice continually encourages my body and mind to relax. It helps me release the tight and stiff fascia that I have come to live with as a by-product of the CRPS. Sometimes I even doze off during a class, but I never worry about what others are doing around me with their movements—I listen to my body.

Craniosacral therapy has definitely helped me with the spasms and stiffness. Even today my physical therapist uses some of the techniques with me when it appears necessary. It is important to tune in and understand that it's possible to release some of that taut connective tissue. I researched and learned about the Feldenkrais Method and decided to go to some classes. It is almost a form of neurological reeducation for the body.

Although nothing is a quick fix, of course, over time and with a lot of dedication, I have experienced tremendous benefits from all these therapies. One therapy or doctor seems to lead me to another, and although at times I have only taken baby steps toward wellness, it is worth the effort and time!

Jill's Story

I was diagnosed in April 2003 as having what one of my doctors called a "severe case" of CRPS. I actually was initially misdiagnosed with plantar fasciitis and was facing surgery in my foot. It all started when I was coaching soccer in the fall of 2002, and my right foot became very painful over the course of two months. By February, I could no longer work and was in excruciating pain, which was mirroring over to my left foot.

On March 25 at 2:30 AM I was awakened by shooting, throbbing, intense (level ten) pain running up both my legs from my feet, all the way to my heart area. I ended up in the hospital emergency room with pain throbbing back and forth between my chest and feet. My symptoms changed in May, when my hands started to suffer tremors and electrical shocks. The shocks relaxed my muscles, and I would drop things. The pain spread throughout my body to my eyes, hands, tongue, and chest area around my heart. My eyes began to spasm, almost as when the picture on a TV set goes into horizontal lines. Or I saw negatives of positive images, similar to the negative of a photograph. I couldn't drive until I could get this under control.

Since then I've gone from a wheelchair to crutches to a cane to now walking on my own. I was originally on all sorts of pain medications, opioids, and antidepressants; I was up to seven types of medications for the pain. Now I'm down to four, and soon it will be three.

I've learned biofeedback, which has helped me enormously with dealing with sudden bursts of pain from my chest. Because I took a chance and my doctor recommended I take Thalidomide to stop the spreading of the CRPS into my eyes and mouth, my eye symptoms have decreased significantly (over 80 percent) and my tongue symptoms by 100 percent. I can drive because the spasm is very light, and my eyes only *feel* the spasms.

Overall, the treatment I've followed has included medications, biofeedback, massage therapy, acupuncture, five nerve blocks in my epidural lumbar region, two sympathetic nerve blocks for my right foot, and five epidural thoracic nerve blocks for my chest. I started out using hydrocodone, Lidoderm patches, amitriptyline, alprazolam, Protonix, and Paxil. Now I'm down to biofeedback, swimming four to five times a week, nerve blocks, and 2,400 mg of Neurontin a day.

Music therapy for CRPS should be considered. Listening to certain music helped me find the courage to say, "No way—I'm not going to live like this." Each person probably has a personal preference about music; my favorite was the soundtrack to the movie *The Lord of the Rings: Fellowship of the Rings*. I used the character Frodo as my guide and imagined myself working just as hard as he did to go through the worst possible adventure (in my case, CRPS) and come out of it.

I plan on going back to work (I teach art in grades five through eight), and I'm so encouraged and hopeful about that. I realize I will have bad days, but I want to think of them as days to remember how bad I was and how great I am now.

I believe my doctors, my husband and family, a massage therapist, acupuncture, and my attitude got me where I am today. I'm happy to say other people can do this, too. You have to have an open mind and believe that you must try every avenue in order to find what works for you. Yes, this requires *hard work,* but isn't a life of activity worth it?

Making Progress

Despite all these support systems and practices to help you along the way, it's crucial to remember that the path of healing tends to zigzag. I still repeat to myself countless times the reassuring mantra of "two steps forward, one step back," with which my occupational therapist used to counsel me as I hung on her every word with tears in my eyes. Once I learned that "truth," I focused on this course and its peculiar nature rather than the final end. To arm yourself against this tug-of-war between progress and setbacks, set your mind on the process of healing, step-by-step. Eventually, you'll find your rhythm.

Why is this so crucial? Think of the last time your physical sensations scared you, surprised you, or snuck right back up when you thought you had moved on to a higher level of functioning. Panic, pity, and emotional collapse can occur within three minutes, followed by tears. Not far behind come automatic thoughts, such as, "I'm broken, and I thought I was better!" Or, "I'm broken for life!" Fight this despair with your very heart and focus on the *process*. Don't give in to these lightning-quick assumptions and remember that we all—with CRPS or not—are works in progress. Try to think of all the top athletes who bandage themselves up before a competition; everyone must take care, take precautions. We *all* may need a little help some time or another, but this does not mean we are innately damaged.

In the interim, try to temper your expectations for becoming perfectly complication-free, and instead focus on your day-to-day healthful practices. Doing so will help you better occupy your mind and keep you focused on improved function.

Dynamite Distractions

Hey, you deserve a little bit of fun now and then. In fact, it can be just what the doctor ordered.

With CRPS, getting well is a full-time job—and you can easily risk becoming a workaholic. Distraction from your pains, both physical and emotional, can become your new best friend—and can be considered a form of therapy in and of itself. While sometimes it is impossible to do anything but be virtually petrified in agony, doing your best to keep going, keep thinking, and keep learning is a necessity.

What is meant by distraction? Absolutely anything that engages your heart, mind, or funny bone and pulls them elsewhere—out of pain's grasp. Unfortunately, as many of you well know, the old ways of being and enjoying yourself might not be possible right now. John the dancer and Sophie the knitter are now left to find new identities—as well as new methods of seeking pleasure in life. This can be devastating, and, yes, you are justified in passing through a grieving period over this. However, the therapeutic importance of distracting and pleasing yourself—quickly—is more urgent than how you used to do things or what hobbies you've lost. At this very moment, try to focus on the *opportunity* to learn new diversions and hold off on mourning the loss of your favorite hobbies. Consider these losses temporary, but rather than waiting around for them to return, seize the chance to amuse yourself in a new way. Better yet, relish the notion of participating in something with no pressure to do it well.

In this chapter, you'll find an array of options and diversions to help you live, love, and laugh larger than your pain, as well as a few mental exercises I use to upstage panic or bitterness. Use these as a launching ground for your own tricks and fill in the spaces allowed for you to customize your distraction strategy.

Remember: While you might read about activities that you currently cannot engage in, I guarantee you will find others in the list, suggested by other CRPS patients, which you will be able to pick up and try. Perhaps you were a very physical person before, engaging in sports, and now your creativity and intellect will ignite as you participate in a new hobby. Or maybe you can find a new way to engage in an old, familiar hobby or activity, as Coleen's story illustrates later in the chapter. Maybe you loved to play piano before but can now take up early morning hikes instead. Let your enjoyment be a form of meditation; engage your mind and your spirit in this discovery and let them soar high above your physical circumstances.

Comedy

At my worst times, I have fixated on humor and waited anxiously for each chance to release a cascade of belly laughs. Numerous studies have focused on the benefits of humor therapy on disease outcome, and in the case of CRPS, "anything goes" if it can make you laugh at the world and yourself. How far will you go in pushing your own humor limits? This is a process that you'll feel out over time, but it requires dedication to make laughing a habit.

It is often said that the best humor comes out of pain. I have found humor in the strangest of places and acted on it, no matter how bizarre or dark it would have seemed to me if I'd done this years ago. For example, I was surprised to find that putting together a mini fashion show to parade my new adaptive clothing line, equipment, and sleep gear actually lightened up the vain side of myself that was crying over such changes. And everyone was impressed by the hefty, padded braces that keep my wrists and elbows straight, an outfit that earned me the title of "Robocop." Finding these off-the-wall "pockets" where you and your family can connect will help to remove the overtly scary, "medical" feel of these strange devices that have entered your life.

Eventually, I found that one of my best therapeutic times was spent with a friend who I could make laugh—rather than vice versa. Explore your sense of humor and find what touches you— whether it is the local improvisation group in your town, stand-up comedians on video or cable, twisted in-family humor, or light-hearted films. Comedy just may become your own personal "faith" of sorts. Here are a few films to get you started, but you can also make your own list:

Ten Videos for Guaranteed Laughs

Anchorman

Best in Show

Chris Rock, Bring the Pain

A Fish Called Wanda

The Full Monty

Legally Blonde

Love and Death

The Royal Tenenbaums

The Best of Saturday Night Live [any year, any version]

Saving Grace

Questions to Consider

What are some of your favorite funny-bone films?

_____

_____

What are some stories or memories that always make you laugh?

_____

_____

Who do you think is one of the funniest people on earth?

_____

_____

Miscellaneous Brain Candy

When was the last time you took inventory of the latest board games for adults? Do you spend most of your time reading about CRPS online, or do you make visits to other sites just for mental pleasure? During my first few months at the doctor's office, I could not bear to speak with other spouses, parents, and patients about all the uncertainties of CRPS; instead, I buried my head in books and magazines discussing foreign cultures, silly stories, and other offbeat trivia. I felt a sense of triumph in knowledge of abstract issues and far-off peoples' different approaches to handling serious life issues. At dinner tables when I felt the pain would blast me off into insanity, my aunt and I would play a simple game of geography [the game in which the first person names a place (country, city, state) and the next person then has to name another place that begins with the last letter in the place named] to keep me engaged and on track.

Involving your brain in problem-solving projects that are un-related to your life issues can be an engaging release—and even, in some instances, be a great new way to revive communication and participate in a project with your loved ones amid a stressful time. Even now, playing charades with my husband and close friends redirects my attention; this gives them a break as well.

Here's a run-through of a few areas to look to solely for pleasure. They temporarily pull your attention away from the pain-anxiety rumination cycle. Add your own ideas to this list and make "brain candy" a regular therapy.

Games

Celebrity Head	Cranium	Risk
Charades	Geography	Taboo

Websites

Brain Candy—a site for mental exercises, quotes, wordplays and jokes: www.corsinet.com/braincandy

Dave Letterman's Top-Ten Lists—quick humor lists: www.cbs.com/shows/late_show/top_ten

Jokes and Comics—free web content: www.jokes.com and www.gocomics.com

Mental Floss—a magazine to engage your curiosity: www.mentalfloss.com

News of the Weird—a report of true and strange stories: www.newsoftheweird.com

The Onion—a satirical American news magazine: www.theonion.com

Flipboard—a well-curated news aggregator/newsreader: www.flipboard.com

Others to personalize your list:

_____

_____

_____

_____

Emotional Release

You may be keeping negative emotions at bay so as to better function day-to-day, but it is positive and therapeutic to find a safe place for you to cry as well. Releasing those emotions can clear out your mind, body, and spirit. That said, a sad, poignant, or simply moving film or book offers substance and something to cry along with—and at the same time provides something to weep about beyond yourself.

Sound fun? Perhaps *fun* is not the correct word, but sad, sensitive films can actually provide entertainment and therapeutic catharsis that I urge you to try from time to time. Such films can both speak to your pains and pull you out of your universe to recognize and share another's sorrows. You may actually find watching these films uplifting and find yourself feeling thankful that you don't face the same challenges as the characters!

Though my experience with CRPS has made me sensitive enough to cry along with just about any film, I've searched the world over for some poignant movies to start with. Grab a tissue and stream online (or pop the following into your DVD player):

Ten Poignant Films

Less than Zero	*Requiem for a*	*Terms of Endearment*
Love Story	*Dream*	*The Thief* [Russian]
My Life Without Me	*Schindler's List*	*12 Years a Slave*
Out of Africa	*Sophie's Choice*	

You can also make your own list.

Music

Music can often touch places in us that nothing else can reach. True, you may have already changed your repertoire of tunes because the old favorites are now too "jumpy," or perhaps you played a musical instrument and must retire your hands for a while.

Again, dropping one area leaves doors open for another. How can you explore and fine-tune your new song?

I found the soundtrack to *Notre Dame de Paris* to be lyrical, gentle, touchingly beautiful, and soothingly distant from my own situation. I could feel along with the music without any words sparking ideas in my head that would make me think (and thus worry). I needed to place my mind elsewhere, in a zone that allowed feelings and moods without words. Familiar music was already packed with memories and symbols, and I needed new material to suit my state; finally, I had the patience to try it during all my time spent resting. Cesoria Evora, a Brazilian singer, has a smooth, calm but moving selection of music, and Habib Koité creates a rhythmic, uplifting atmosphere with his music. Here are some ways you can move beyond your standard uses for music:

Explore world music. Smooth bossa nova, Middle-Eastern music, French love songs, African chants, uplifting yoga music, Ayurvedic music, ambient and trance music, and lounge and meditation music are all available online, at music stores, or even from the library. Try www.newworldmusic.com or www.di.fm to start.

Become a lyrics expert. Learn the words to your favorite tunes or explore new songs and songwriters whose words might touch you more now. Start at www.pandora.com or www.lyrics.com, both of which play the songs that are transcribed on the sites. You can also find many online music-lover groups at www.facebook.com.

Learn an instrument. The flute and the guitar seem to be the easiest and most portable instruments that don't produce an overwhelming amount of vibration. Use your local paper or musical instrument store to find either a teacher or a friend willing to come to your house and offer lessons. Or you might try teaching yourself guitar without being able to read music: Grab a simple chords book and start with guitar "tablature" to various surprisingly simple songs (available in music stores, at the library, online, at www.all tabs.com, or via various guitar tab applications you can download on your phone). You'll find that many of your favorite tunes use only two or three chords.

Sing! The benefits of singing have recently been compared to those of practicing yoga, as the diaphragmatic breathing encourages relaxation. Sing when you feel well, sing when you are struggling, and—depending on how mobile you are—look into finding a chorus or other group and sing with others.

Creating Sanctuary

CRPS might have derailed your original life plans, but by going off-track, you can seize this time to explore the road less traveled. If you're not in step with the so-called standard reality of daily activities and responsibilities rumbling outside your window, this is your chance to construct your own reality. I've always believed that we each create our own reality—what we perceive to be reality and how it is treating us—in our lives. And we each are empowered mentally to conceive of the most nurturing, joyous, and colorful reality that we want.

I surround myself with colors, flowers, and inspiring quotes. I do this because I know my heart and mind need as much encouragement as possible. The colors and flowers represent growth, health, and vibrancy—traits I feel I lost with CRPS and am now in the process of regaining. When I feel bad, my environment supports me. Even though my hands are burning, my retreat from daily activities means I return to a resting spot where positive words, smiling colors, and strong green plants envelop me and my psyche. Then I return to activity as soon as I see improvement in physical symptoms—because my spirit and mind remain positive and intact in the interim. You, too, can focus on creating a nurturing environment for yourself. In fact, it can develop into a hobby, an ongoing process. The following are a few ideas to get you started:

Project One: A Personal Shrine

Take a plain photo frame, easily found at a craft store, and use glue, paints, buttons, fabric, shells, colored stones, or miniature tiles to decorate and personalize it. Place a photo of a special memory or a person you love inside the frame. Better yet, see if you can find materials to make your own picture frame, such as cardboard, plastic, or wood. Using a moment to express your imagination in something joyous can fill you with compassion, patience, hope, and remembrance of things that bring you pleasure.

Place your personal shrines around your home, especially in places where you practice meditation or need a reminder to "keep going."

Project Two: Softness and Scents

Whether you're the most feminine female or rough-edged man, a soft, comfortable place that suits your body can mean the world to you during a difficult moment. Likewise, a soothing scent that you associate with that place can prove relaxing. Experiment with different fabrics and the softness or density of pillows to suit your needs, along with scented candles that match how you feel and how you'd like to feel at any given moment. When your tastes change, allow yourself to bend with them. Oftentimes simply focusing on this practice of creating sanctuary for times of need can give you a feeling of sanctuary in itself.

Arts and Crafts

People who never before touched a paintbrush or sketchbook have developed their artistic sides after the onset of a pain condition. Art includes so many different types of media that even seasoned artists can change the types of movements and materials they work with to better adapt to CRPS's effects. If your strength is challenged, you can switch from woodworking to gentle watercolor painting; likewise, if this is your first venture into arts and crafts, you may find release and expression of yourself simply through particular colors and free movements with finger painting. Using a different hand or foot and developing its muscular control—or taking artistic advantage of this lack of control—can be engaging options.

You can use your projects for the immediate pleasure and involvement they allow or to produce useful things, such as gifts or decorations. Consider the following media:

- beadwork and jewelry making
- calligraphy
- collage making
- crayons
- knitting and crocheting
- mosaics with glass
- paints
- pastels
- tile work
- weaving and sewing

Check your local crafts store (Michael's, for example) for a sampling of materials and booklets to guide you. A wonderful book for nurturing or reframing your artistic side is *The Encyclopedia of Craft Projects for the First Time*.

Questions to Consider

What do you consider "beautiful"?

_____

_____

_____

What textures and colors do you enjoy? Which make you feel comforted, calm, or cozy?

_____

_____

_____

Art Project One: Color Exploration

Imagine inhaling a colored mist or a light that comforts and relaxes you. Let this color become the basis for your exploration. You can paint, draw, or just use finger paints to push beyond your normal boundaries and delve into the essence of this calm. Sometimes when I am unable to concentrate on much else besides nerve sensations in my right arm, I finger paint a calming color with my left; it enables me to enter a "flow" experience for a short bit and tune everything else out as a form of meditation. After years of doing this in layers, I have some abstract art pieces to show for it.

Art Project Two: The Nerve Circus

Do you have a pain circus going on? Are you shocked by how interrelated your nerves are throughout your body? Use the following mental and visual exercise to look at your situation with the "big top" approach: Try to express your experience of pain by portraying (by paint, marker, charcoal, glitter, glued objects, etc.) the circus tent, the performers involved, and even the audience being affected by your condition. For different forms of pain, you can visualize flamethrowers and knife swallowers. Risky trapeze acts can represent the unpredictability of CRPS's effects and the uncertainty you feel about the future.

Creating a coherent image of all that is occurring can offer a sense of release from its chaos. You may even be able to use it to explain your health situation and body sensations to your loved ones, or even have your family members help you create it. This artistic metaphor may carry a lighter, more tolerable tone for both you and your loved ones.

Art Project Three: Scribble-Blot Spontaneity

Scribbling with your nondominant or unaffected hand can provide access to undiscovered, free-association pockets of your personality. Rather than limiting your mastery of arts, this relinquishing of control can help you expand and capitalize on spontaneity in your personal expression. You can also use blots of paints on a page, fold the page in half, and develop the image you see in the blot into a feeling, a person, the birth process, and so on with paint, pen, pastels, or charcoal. Or dip a string or piece of yarn into ink and liberate yourself from expectations, moving the string across paper to your liking. Involving your brain in this unusual practice can be meditative, leaving you feeling balanced and reinvigorated with possibility. It may allow you to dip into an area that otherwise is too confusing to tap into just yet.

Check in with the Masters

Try developing an interest in contemporary art or art history, and you'll find many artists have used their genius to express their own experiences of physical and emotional pain—as well as hope and inspiration. Read up on the masters! Look around at local work that talks to you, find a favorite artist, and believe in their work as a beautiful way to express your own feelings. Bookstores and libraries are full of colorful art books to start with; keep a large, colorful book that you enjoy in close reach in your home for times when you need to switch mindsets and combat a despairing moment. You don't need to be a jetsetter or an academic—or even know how to paint—in order to appreciate great art! You might even want to try volunteering at a local art center or artists' alliance to seek out new, stimulating input and to combat loneliness.

Nature Hiking

If you are able to walk outside, a brisk walk through nature is one of the best ways to release anxiety while regaining perspective and connectivity to the world around you. Forget notions of whether you were an "outdoorsy" person before and simply try it. Start off slowly and familiarize yourself with the terrain in order to prevent falls or further injury.

Rather than having a distance or height goal in mind, focus on your surroundings and decide which elements of the hike you most enjoy. Do you enjoy examining the different trees and flowers? Animals? Can you find peace in listening to the natural sounds of the forest and the air around you—or do you prefer listening to a relaxing or inspiring song or audiobook on your iPod? Do you need to go on a long hike, or is ten minutes sufficient for you in the outdoors? Do you like watching the sun rise? Set? Is this something you find more rewarding in solitude, or could this be something you'd enjoy with others?

Forget the stereotypical hiker; each person derives pleasure and meaning differently from this venture. Pull on a pair of sturdy sneakers or hiking boots (don't hesitate just because someone needs to help you tie them), find a well-known, leafy passageway, and test out a trek.

A great trail and hiking book to assist you is *Backpacker's Start-Up: A Beginner's Guide to Hiking and Backpacking* by Doug Werner. Also try picking up a guide to trees and plants that are found in your local area. This may pose a new type of challenge to you in your surroundings.

Read Sherri's story to see how one CRPS patient is using the goal of an extended hiking trip abroad to stay inspired and encouraged.

*S*herri's Story

I was diagnosed with CRPS in 1993. I have had numerous knee surgeries on my left knee since I was twelve years old. I had six surgeries prior to being diagnosed with RSD and two since being diagnosed. I was diagnosed after hitting my bad knee on the side of my desk one afternoon at work. Considering the major surgeries I had already gone through, I was shocked at the amount of debilitating pain I was enduring just due to bumping my leg.

From 1993 to 1998, I endured almost every medication and procedure imaginable, including being hospitalized with an epidural block for ten days at a time and living on morphine around the clock for a year. Even though I was diagnosed almost immediately, it was determined that due to the improper mechanics of my left leg, which was causing ongoing trauma with use, it would be next to impossible for the CRPS to go into remission. Some of my surgeries included having my kneecap removed, having all of my thigh muscles transplanted, etc.

In 1996 I finally had to go on long-term disability, as the CRPS had traveled up my entire left side. If I had to walk or be on my feet for any length of time, I had to use a wheelchair. I was in a full-leg brace and using a cane as well. I couldn't sit for any length of time and had suffered a tremendous amount of atrophy on my left side.

In 1998 my pain physician and I decided to try having a spinal cord stimulator implanted and see if that would improve my pain level and functionality. As soon as the stimulator was implanted, I could actually put my knee on the operating table and allow it to be touched. At first the pain relief was sporadic, but as scar tissue formed around the electrode in my spine an amazing thing happened. *It worked.* It relieved about 60 to 70 percent of my pain.

I only needed to continue to take pain medication at night in order to sleep. It was exciting to be able to go out and buy my first pair of jeans in over five years and to even shave my legs! I learned to meditate and do tai chi for people with disabilities, both of which I continue to do every day. I also found a wonderful pain counselor who helped me to let go of the things I could no longer do and helped me to discover a new life and accept my limitations. I went back to work full-time in 1999 and have been improving ever since. I am already using my second spinal cord stimulator battery.

I am very lucky though to be considered a "virtual employee" of American Express. I work from home full-time. This allows me the flexibility to do whatever I need to do to remain healthy and stay as pain-free as possible. It is hard to maintain enough balance in my life to stay relatively pain-free, but when I consider the alternative, there is no choice. Since my left side doesn't have an "accurate thermostat," a change in the weather (in temperature or an increase in humidity) can be extremely devastating. Sometimes I just keep moving through the pain of a flare-up, knowing it will pass.

I continue to remain fairly active. I walk two to three miles a day, five to six days a week. Considering I was wheelchair bound for a while, this is a huge improvement for me. Things are going so well that I have recently decided to begin planning a trip. It's a personal journey to reflect on how far I've come and a reminder that I can continue to live with CRPS and still reach goals and have a lifetime of personal accomplishments and good memories. I am planning to hike the Highlands of Scotland during the summer of 2005. I am giving myself enough time to train for the hiking. The trip consists of day hikes anywhere from seven to twelve miles. It is a guided trip and will last a week, with five of those days being hiking days. This might not sound like a challenge for a healthy individual, but for me this will be one of the biggest challenges I have ever faced besides being diagnosed with CRPS.

Gardening: A New Slant

You do not have to have a green thumb in order to add some green to your life. Rather, you can consider gardening to be any practice of honoring organic life, growth, and bloom. With the specter of loss, dysfunction, and biological abnormality looming over your CRPS experience, keeping in touch with positive, dynamic forces of nature can be inspiring and supportive. Being able to make something else grow can reintroduce the notion of wonder into your life—especially if you are the one in charge of this life force.

There are many ways to create a sense of garden and verdure, depending on where you live, your physical abilities, and your family.

Plotted. Plant a bit of a real garden outside. Remember to start slowly and pace yourself to prevent unfinished projects caused by pain interruptions. Try just planting a few low-maintenance plants at first, such as chamomile, violet, or snow-in-summer as ground coverings; aster or daylily as perennials; and rosemary, rose, or mahonia as shrubs. Start simply with a wildflower or herbal lawn seed mix to add some color to the environment within your reach.

Gardening is a great means for working together and connecting with your friends, children, or neighbors. Make a daily practice of spending time in your garden and be mindful of these other living elements. Rest on a stool that can be left in your garden and try a breathing exercise outside.

Potted. Keep a few potted plants (e.g., basil) on your windowsill. This can be a very low-maintenance endeavor and can include just a few elements of nature that you care for, smell, control the growth of, and even use. Consider these wonders every time you pass your plants.

Papered. A great project for your children is to build a paper/crafts garden. They can cut out paper "garden" figures in the forms of tulips, tomatoes, watermelon, and other lush, bright images and decorate a relaxing, cheery corner of your home with these cut-outs. This can be an ongoing project for you and can provide a new way to interact with your children, engage them, and help keep your home positively oriented toward nature and growth. When you're not feeling well, draw your children in with a project for the garden. Tell them that you "could really use a bright new flower," and your children—rather than feeling helpless or left alone—can feel useful and involved by adding a bright new addition to the home garden and making you feel better.

Imagined. If none of these options are available, remember that one of the most powerful gardens you can manage is the one in your imagination. Fill it with positive people, experiences you're thankful for, hope, and opportunities that may come—all the things that bathe your soul in sunlight and make you bloom as a person. You will always have at least a few flowers in this garden: you, your hope, your spirit, and your compassion. Escape there and add to it—not only in times of need, but as an exercise in normal daydreaming.

For plant encyclopedias, ideas, and photographs do an online search or try www.theplantencyclopedia.org.

Bird-Watching

You may have never considered this activity before, but it can offer an opportunity to focus on physical beings other than yourself, a new contemplation of nature, a study of beautiful creatures, and a very accessible activity from even your bedroom window. You will find many online and in-person groups that gather to talk about bird-watching; this might be a great way to communicate with others and feel connected, even while participating in a largely private experience. Why not try an outing in a nearby nature reserve or nature center—or consider a project involving your children to set up a bird feeder outside your window?

To get started, try *Birding for Beginners* by Sheila Buff, or *Backyard Birding* by Terence Lindsay and R. G. Turner. Or dive right into the *National Geographic Field Guide to Birds* for your continent or region.

Photography

Photography possesses a wondrous relationship with time, mood, and memory—and can be another way for you to focus on the world around you or creatively provide testament to your current state of mind. Not only does technology increasingly cater to the camera user's needs, but books and the Internet enable you to learn about photography at your own private pace.

Whether you have picked up the camera before or this is your first time using one, your camera can offer a different perspective or slant on your reality. Do you wish to beautify and soften what you see and feel around you? Do you wish to photograph the people who mean the most to you, to take a closer look at nature that comforts you, or to document your feelings and moods amid CRPS as a form of journaling? Whatever aspect you wish to focus on, photography can provide—literally—a different lens with which to look at your life, your self, others, and your pain.

Whenever your pain or anxiety becomes too much, picking up the camera may provide a change of pace and a place to channel your energies. You can join a group or chat online; you can even share your work with others.

For inspiration with fantastic shots, information on each type of camera and how it works, the history of photography, and numerous links to books and online courses, start by looking at the websites for the American Museum of Photography (www.photo graphymuseum.com) or the New York Institute of Photography (www.nyip.com).

Questions to Consider

How do you see yourself differently since your pain started? Experiment with auto snapshots.

_____

_____

_____

How do you see others differently? Can you capture your unique perspective with the camera?

_____

_____

_____

Which images or figures seem powerful to you right now?

_____

_____

_____

_____

Which images give you strength, make you smile or leave you awe-struck?

_____

_____

_____

Traveling Inward

When your days are filled with pain, finding meaning in your life becomes more important than ever. Take this time to explore what values, ideologies, and spiritual notions you believe in. You may have had a fuzzy or even a very solid idea of faith before this challenge, but you may find you have to rearrange or delve further into the question of faith to suit your current needs. You may believe in a specific organized religion, you may believe in creativity and music, or you may believe in certain social causes. Test them and learn more about approaches available to you for living your life. You may find you want to mix-and-match various ideas and notions to create your own personal faith.

Grab an old book that presented an idea with which you once strongly identified, or turn to regular readings of familiar religious texts, whether it is the Bible, the Koran, the Torah, the Bhagavad Gita, or some other text. Or bridge the gap between daily life and traditional religion with the following insightful books that can provide ideas for rethinking yourself, your body, and your health. These books touch on spirituality, pain, holistic health, and psychology.

Books for Introspection
Being Peace by Thich Nhat Hanh
Beyond the Relaxation Response by Herbert Benson, MD
Full Catastrophe Living by Jon Kabat-Zinn, PhD

The Impossible Just Takes a Little Longer by Art Berg
Letting Go of the Person You Used to Be by Lama Surya Das
A Life Larger than Pain by Erv Hinds, MD
Solitude: A Return to the Self by Anthony Storr

Questions to Consider

What do you want to learn about yourself?

_____

_____

_____

What do you find most mysterious about life right now?

_____

_____

_____

How do you see your emotions and beliefs interacting with your physical health?

_____

_____

_____

Would you be open to new ways of thinking about life?

_____

_____

_____

_____

What type of encouragement would fill a gap in your life or nurture faith in yourself right now?

_____

_____

_____

_____

Traveling Outward

As CRPS tends to isolate you, remaining connected to the world beyond your medical case poses a challenge. While some old links may be severed through this experience, you can also find joy and meaning in new ones. Volunteering can provide a way for you to feel useful and to test out your currently diminished/slowly increasing functional abilities in a supportive environment where your efforts will be appreciated. It also can provide you with an opportunity to try out a new career direction you might wish to pursue or to explore an interest you never had the courage or time to address before. Whatever volunteer activity you choose, you will exercise your ability to concentrate and remember information, a skill that might have greatly declined during the recent phases of your illness.

Six months after developing CRPS, I started volunteering just two hours a week as a Spanish interpreter alongside a doctor at a Hispanic charity clinic. Those two hours were shaky the first few times, but I felt safe around this doctor—and found I absolutely treasured our chats and stories we shared alongside the interpreting work. Without my ever expecting it, he (and this volunteer position) served as my link to the outside world and became a new friend as well. I looked forward to those two hours each week as a symbol of my feeling useful, empowered, and in great company. I knew how to question patients about the types of pain they were experiencing, because my own experience made me understand how many types exist. While I still could not use my arms, my language skills were appreciated, and I felt a side of my personality that was dormant at the time—my brain—take the lead over my body. Soon those two hours turned into four hours, and then six; I was able to use this volunteer experience to explore Spanish interpreting as a career alternative in researching options following my prior typing-intensive career at a communications firm.

Is there a certain cause with which you strongly identify? Can you imagine something with which you can get lightly involved? Check your local library for postings, or search the Action Without Borders website at www.idealist.org.

Last-Resort Reality-Check Exercise, or "Misery Loves Company"

Sometimes I just don't want to channel my energy positively. When I'm too filled with despair or bitterness, even yoga or meditation may not always answer my needs; that's when I try another approach: a reality check. In this exercise, I think of five people who have been dealt a difficult blow and who are suffering extraordinarily at this very moment.

It does not have to be someone known personally, but make your images of them as detailed and realistic as possible: a child who has lost his legs via a bomb or a friend who has lost his fiancée in a car crash. I focus on the details and emotions of such images to remind myself that I'm not alone, separate from the rest of the world in my suffering—and that our fortunes are so unpredictable and liable to change from day to day. The exercise may seem morbid, but it eliminates any jealousy I may have toward others' apparent ease in the world, provides a larger grasp of the world to which I belong, and even offers a bit of hope in the unknown of tomorrow.

Keep a Distraction Quick List

When you have an "off-duty" moment, one in which you are able to think about and engage in things you love, try to think about what always makes you smile or something that makes you feel curious, deliciously soothed, or challenged. Jot down your ideas—a website, a game, a favorite columnist, or a comedian—and keep this list handy at all times.

Granted, there's always "something to do" for your health, self-care, and daily life responsibilities. But take a break daily to have a little bit of fun. Again: Fun is a therapeutic blessing. It gets different parts of your mind running, offers pleasure, and exercises your brain. Any time spent revisiting your old lighthearted feelings or generating new thoughts outside of the pain box is beneficial.

Coleen, whose story ends this chapter, has been fortunate enough to be able to return to some of the extremely physical activities she loves. Her inspiring story highlights the importance of continuing to thrive—even in the face of RSD/CRPS—by finding and living one's passions.

Coleen's Story

I have had CRPS for about fifteen years now. I was in a very nasty head-on car accident twenty-one years ago. I broke my back and pelvis. I was paralyzed from the waist down. I was in the hospital for about three months. As time went by I got to the point where I could walk with a walker, then crutches, then a cane, then a brace, and now with no assistance.

I damaged a lot of nerves, as you could expect. During the first five to six years after the accident I went through four foot surgeries trying to correct the way I walk. I walk on the outside of my left foot due to the nerve damage. Sometime during those foot surgeries I developed CRPS.

I do all the things many people who have CRPS do. I take narcotics, I have sought counseling, I see a doctor at a pain clinic on a regular basis, and I have gone through—and continue to go through—nerve blocks. However, the things that I do that most people with CRPS don't do are play softball, ride horses, and rope cows. I am the captain of my women's ice hockey team, and I also play in a men's ice hockey league. I also go to the gym three to five times a week.

Many of my teammates know the challenges I face to even get my skate on my foot. Many of my teammates do not even know my history. Most of the time I try to just keep that to myself. I do wear quite a large orthotic to be able to play hockey. So sometimes when another player sees the brace they ask why I wear it. If people ask me about the "interesting" way I skate, I tell them what happened. What they say when they hear the story is almost always the same: "I would have never guessed that you had any physical challenges!"

Trust me, some days it takes everything I have just to get my skates on, let alone go out and play! I guess the thing that I have found that helps me to live as close to an ordinary life as possible is I've always agreed with the saying, "Everyone needs three things: someone to love, something to do, and something to look forward to." Ice hockey, among other things, covers all three of those things for me! I truly believe that if each CRPS patient fulfills those three things, it is easier to cope with this nasty disease. The more we as patients can stay active and participate in our own "passions," the easier it is to cope with CRPS.

Help for the Helper: A Chapter for Caregivers

Being a CRPS caregiver is one of the most difficult balancing acts around. Somehow you must understand your loved one's condition intimately while also providing him or her with a bridge to the outside world and its demands. Since CRPS is such an isolating condition, the caregiver must check in and guard against burnout.

Knowing how to address your loved one's needs, if you're both new to CRPS, can take some time and guesswork. Likewise, so too can the practice of drawing the line between giving yourself to others and keeping your own self whole and healthy. Many have said that going through this experience is the only way to truly design your customized rules of engagement. However, using knowledge as a framework for approaching your loved one and being prepared for certain emotions and reactions that you both will stumble across can help you realize that you're not alone on this path.

This chapter is for brave caregivers needing support. It is also for people who are not direct caregivers but who wish to be better friends and helpers to those more involved. The more *everyone* knows, the smaller the burden placed on any one person to be an expert or Superman. Let's begin by outlining a few of the challenges involved in your role.

Understanding the Patient

Why is it that your loved one can feel capable and lighthearted for a few hours—and be stricken with disabling pain the next few? Gauging what he or she can do, can concentrate on, and can offer to you emotionally is a strenuous guessing game that can leave you breathless, perplexed, and feeling out of control. Just when you think you've identified the patterns, activities, and emotions that set off your loved one's pain, CRPS throws you another curveball. Let's try to break down the game.

By nature of the condition, CRPS tends to fluctuate in intensity both in the course of healing and as a chronic illness. What may register as two steps forward one week can also include one step backward the next; likewise, your loved one's general well-being can chronically bounce up and down. The key is understanding that this process is normal, reducing the height of fluctuations to a more steady state, and perceiving just how sensitive the CRPS patient is to a variety of factors.

Gauging the Pain

First of all, the use of pain-intensity scales can help you and your loved one understand the type and degree of pain she or he is experiencing on a given day. To gauge the intensity of CRPS pain, take a look at the McGill Pain Index from McGill University and developed by Melzer and Torgerson in Figure 2. Created in 1971, this index illustrates types and levels of pain for various conditions, presenting a coherent consistency in various aspects of pain that doctors use around the world—even though pain is still an intensely personal experience. Crucially, you'll see causalgia listed extremely high on the scale; causalgia, which is complex regional pain syndrome type 2 (CRPS 2), is the Latin term to denote burning pain, found in both CRPS types 1 (RSD) and 2 (causalgia).

Another way for you to discuss pain levels on a day-to-day basis is by using a scale of 1 to 10. The Joint Commission now requires hospitals and other health-care facilities to measure pa-

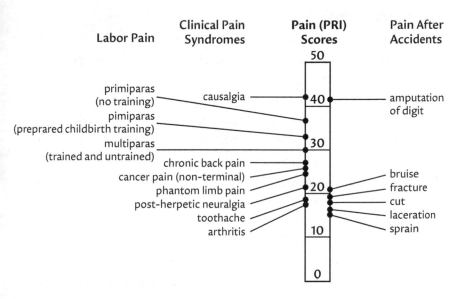

FIGURE 2. The McGill Pain Index
(Reprinted from *Textbook of Pain,* edited by Patrick D. Wall and
Ronald Melzack, pp. 339–45, ©1999, with permission from Elsevier)

tients' pain on an expanded scale of 0 to 10. You can interpret pain levels as follows:

0–1: I have no pain at all or I can barely notice it.

2–3: I have a little pain, but I'm comfortable.

4–5: I have pain. I feel uncomfortable when I'm resting or active. It is not too bad, but maybe I could feel better.

6–7: I have pain that is always on my mind. I can do things, but it is difficult.

8–9: I have so much pain that I cannot do anything. When I have pain like this, I cannot rest. I can think only about the pain.

10: This is the worst pain I could possibly feel. I cannot stand this pain.

(Adapted from the "Pain Guide" handout distributed to some patients at Columbia Presbyterian Hospital.)

The Elements

Weather is a common complaint in affecting pain levels. Cold, humidity, rain, and particularly changes in barometric pressure often cause increased discomfort—while someone who is not in pain may not even feel the subtle changes taking place outside. Try keeping up-to-date on daily weather to anticipate "needier" days or stress factors. You can encourage your loved one to monitor his or her symptoms in relation to the weather reports and to use the weather guide as one of your dialogue points in expressing needs and pains.

Emotional/Psychological Stressors

Stress, fear, anticipation, and anxiety are colossally common in CRPS, and they are also dangerous cyclical pain perpetrators and exacerbators. Encouraging a sense of peace, calmness, and security about the future—even in light of your very real concerns—can be one of the greatest medical and interpersonal deeds you can do for your loved one. Even if you and your loved one have a right to worry about her situation, your loved one does not have the medical luxury of putting her body through such distress. There is no greater justice than her health, and no display of anxiety is ever justified because in the case of CRPS, additional anxiety may have a negative effect on the patient's health and well-being. This is something to remember for yourself as well. Find new ways to distract or calm your friend or loved one to keep her on track when pain or panic narrows her problem-solving ability. Meditation may be something that not only your loved one but also you partake in—possibly together.

Other Irritants

Vibrations from machines or loud music (especially bass), bumpy car rides, drafts from air conditioners or fans, or loud noises can set off the "pain soldiers" that can march through your loved one's body. You can ease the CRPS patient's anticipatory anxiety and fear of being "a drag" if you, too, become vigilant about these irritants. For example, if you go out for an evening with your loved one and others, try to speak up before the CRPS sufferer has to if you see you'll be sitting below an air-conditioner vent in a restaurant; similarly, suggest alternatives to going out to a loud music club so that the person with CRPS is not left at the club's door, counting how much cash he has for a quiet cab ride home at the last minute.

Certain foods or chemicals, such as caffeine and nitrates, can cause added irritation. Finally, lack of harmony in relationships becomes all the more distressing to CRPS patients at a time when they believe that these relationships are their only lifelines. Try to let petty issues and dramatic escalations fall to the wayside and talk out issues as honestly as possible. Try to utilize this time to delve deeper into your relationship with your loved one and use this as an opportunity to find meaning. Both of you can come out of this experience as more introspective, deeper individuals than you ever imagined possible. There is, actually, no way you couldn't....

Lending a Hand

For those just starting out as caregivers—or if you have too much on your plate—there is a way to make assistance really matter: If you want to offer help, be specific. While telling your friend or loved one "Let me know how I can help" or "Let me know if I can do anything" may include the sincerest of intentions, it's most likely that he will be least likely to reach out when he needs it most. The myriad of things for which he needs help may be overwhelming and difficult to articulate. In addition, deep-seated frustration and shame can also surround the CRPS patient's awareness that he needs help. Not only may he feel a burden in asking for a hand, but he may be downright angry that he has to ask for something he mastered long ago.

You can make it easier for yourself and your friend or loved one by offering to lend a hand with particular tasks, such as providing transportation to a doctor's appointment, going grocery shopping, assisting with paperwork or laundry, or even buckling a seatbelt. Hearing specific offers for assistance greatly relieves the CRPS sufferer's burden of knowing what to ask for and having to ask for it. It can also guide you in brainstorming the various categories in which you can offer aid and clearly define the time commitments needed to finish each task. Finally, being specific can eliminate some of the guesswork that comes along with trying to understand what your loved one is thinking or feeling or needing at a certain time. Any particular, customized actions that tap into his or her world of needs can also help to ease some of the alienation that a person with CRPS (and a caregiver, if there is one) is so often feeling.

Changing Patterns

While you are working to organize a new system for living that accommodates your loved one's needs, you may be frustrated that he or she does not properly respond or direct you while you're "waiting on" him. Perhaps you have drastically changed your life to free up valuable time to assist your friend or family member, and you may feel that she does not recognize and respect your sacrifices. If she did, she would have a plan of what she needs help with—and offer clear instructions.

Your feelings are valid. It's important to understand, however, that the person with CRPS also needs to learn how to plan, verbalize, and direct others to do simple tasks that he or she could do before without thinking. Very few people are accustomed to sitting around and telling someone to carry through their every wish—especially when extreme pain wrangles the sufferer's concentration. Knowing how to utilize help "productively" takes time (for both of you), and, in fact, requires almost a new pattern of thought in the patient.

As a simple example, I used to be a very fast multitasker who focused mentally on one activity while doing two others at the same time. Slowing down this process in order to verbalize it and tell someone to do each activity one at a time required time, practice, and an elimination of my old strategies and thought processes. The simplest tasks, such as telling someone how to put together a sandwich for me, became a lengthy maze through turkey, lettuce, the wheat bread in the bag on the kitchen counter, the Dijon mustard on the upper-right shelf of the refrigerator, and so on. Each ingredient had to be separated from the mix and introduced with additional directions.

This process is a small but illustrative hurdle amid a day of various larger crises and chaos that CRPS can bring. Your loved one is facing a relearning process that requires pulling apart every ingredient of his life and explaining it to another. Amid the pain that tries his patience and blurs his concentration, notions of lost independence and humiliation may flash through his head or pulse within his gut. All of this may be going on—and you're just making a turkey sandwich!

Another obstacle is the fact that your loved one is battling with a changed image of her worth to you and others. Whether or not this image has in fact changed in your eyes, your loved one may be both frightened and angered that she will have to find new ways to be "of value" to you. In my own experience, after being a very independent person, I was aware that friends and family had become the most important things—if not the only things—in my life, while also sensing that my very livelihood depended upon them. I was worried I would lose them at the point when I needed them most. Just when I was not much fun, when I couldn't do the things I did before with them, I was asking them for favors and living on their encouragement—what could I offer them? I assumed that I had to be constantly charming, genial, and walking on eggshells of worthiness as the most bountiful bundle of social grace—now that I could not offer any physical form of activity, independence, or help in our relationship. These types of thoughts can register as insecurity, anger, distance, resistance, and even clinginess in a CRPS patient. To help your loved one overcome this hurdle, remind her that her intrinsic worth is not determined by what she can do or make for you. It seems simple, but voicing it means the world at such a time of precarious self-esteem.

Recalibrating Partnership

Eventually what seems like a loss will become routine and will require much less thought, conscious planning, waiting, and time in general. But then, slowly, in many cases, your friend or loved one will begin to take back responsibilities, carefully creep back into functions, and gently remove weight from your shoulders. This will be another road to travel in undoing learned helplessness, and both of you—together—can celebrate small victories in gained function.

During this time of regaining more balance in the relationship, it is important to take new inventory of what your loved one can do to help you again. It may mean taking back old responsibilities such as laundry, strategizing a different way for him or her to adaptively take charge of certain errands (via mobility services, catalogs, online resources, carpooling), or devising completely new ways in which he or she can offer you assistance. During the long road that you've passed together, from crisis to the more routine maintenance of chronic illness, you have surely learned more about each other's weaknesses and strengths. Making use of the CRPS sufferer's strengths as they resurface can make both of you feel better about your relationship, and reduce the risk for learned helplessness.

Encountering Bumps on the Road to Independence

Once your loved one begins to take back responsibilities, his journey to independence will require your support in a different way. Anger, frustration, and sadness can cloud his recovery route due to the adaptations necessary to do something that was previously easy. Being upset about how much effort is required to achieve the same task—how he cannot fulfill a project the way he could do it before—is a common heartbreak that can last a very long time. Your loved one's emotions might become just as volatile as they were at the onset of illness, due to this challenging frustration in the journey back to regular life.

"What does he want?" you may wonder. "He's better, and yet he's still upset?" Keep in mind that significant relief from pain can still mean much loss and ongoing limitation—just when your loved one has again allowed his expectations to soar as high as anyone else's. Tempering these expectations with realism and feeling gratitude for strides made will take time. Moreover, it is not your job to make him happy and heal all his emotional and psychological wounds. Understanding these wounds can be your part, while an outside professional in psychological counseling is a very necessary aspect of helping a person with CRPS manage these transitions.

Peeking into Each Other's World

Partnership with a loved one in the face of CRPS requires a safe space for clear communication about the changes underway. Equal awareness and respect for both the patient's and the caregiver's experiences and priorities are important in sustaining this new relationship dynamic.

The Patient's World...

Though you may feel your devotion is obvious, the inner and outer struggle your loved one is fighting with CRPS may prevent her from remembering that you are indeed here for her. If she has kept a pain record, diary, artwork, or poetry, ask to see a little of what she has recorded. Learn how she directly interprets this experience to herself—before this information passes through the "translation," explanation, or abridgment phase the person with CRPS feels might be necessary for you to understand. You may be surprised by what you learn, and this new information can help guide you in gauging the emotions, psychology, and physical pain of your loved one.

Even if she refuses and claims it is too personal, you don't have to consider your request to be an unwelcome invasion of privacy. It shows that you care to know *her* side of what it means to have CRPS. Ask again, as sharing one's deepest weaknesses and despair is extremely difficult, and she may not be sure of your dedicated interest. If she still refuses, let it rest; yet be assured that both of you have reached an emotional milestone with this interchange. She will appreciate and feel more unconditionally cared for by knowing that you want to reach out so deeply to her. She might wish to open up more, better trust your capacity for understanding, or offer a glimpse into her private world at a later time.

...And Yours, Too

Likewise, if you're a caregiver, you have your own dreams, worries, anger, and loss tied up in the CRPS experience. Keeping a stiff upper lip and refusing to express the deeply human struggle you are going through is not going to benefit you or your relationship with the CRPS patient in the end. Try walking through how you experience the situation on your own terms—rather than as seen through the patient's eyes. A lot of the methods of recording and expression that a patient can use can also be beneficial and worthwhile for a caregiver. If you have not expressed yourself through some form—artistic or otherwise—it is imperative to do so. See the suggestions offered in Chapters 3 and 7 for keeping a journal or creatively expressing yourself in other ways. Moreover, instead of feeling guilty about having your own negative emotions toward the experience or worrying that you are hurting your loved one, a time will come when sharing your side of the struggle can make you both see eye to eye on how you're a team in this experience. When you ask to see your loved one's interpretation of the experience, also ask if you can show him yours. Who could understand what you're going through better than the patient himself? Revealing your hurts and stresses in a positive manner can also reduce the chances of developing anger toward the patient or toward the fact that you "cannot" or "should not" express such hurts as a caregiver.

In addition, and to voice your experience and alleviate some isolation, you can also participate in the National Caregiver Story Project and contribute your own personal story. This project is sponsored by the National Family Caregivers Association, for which you can find contact information later in this chapter. You can also increase awareness of CRPS by getting the word out about the challenges of caring for this condition.

Since I wrote the first edition of this book, I've gotten married. Learning how to calibrate a dynamic with my husband has been a work in progress, through remission and flare-ups of musculoskeletal pain. I've learned that some acts of independence, taken on my part to spare him, can be costly to the relationship; for example, we've found that having my partner at pivotal medical appointments to witness my experience and frustration firsthand is far preferable to him than emotionally discussing it with me afterward. I feel more understood with him present, and I spare him the postevent emoting. We move on together (or try to).

Using Humor

So okay, laughing about devastating issues can prove extremely sensitive if you don't know where the joker is coming from. Just as subjects such as cancer or ethnic differences can be highly sensitive in certain situations, so too can humor about CRPS make the sufferer feel as if you're making light of the situation. However, in this case, intimate time spent caring for a CRPS patient's needs renders one eligible for truly understanding the moment-to-moment challenges that the patient faces with this condition. While no one can truly experience what another thinks and feels, a sense of understanding between patient and helper can develop and produce a great source of relief, distraction, and perspective: good humor.

It took a while for my family and friends to understand what I was going through, but once we all approached the same level, humor lightened the situation and wove us together in our understanding. I will never forget the time when my best childhood friends reunited to see each other and, primarily, to see how I was doing after months of isolation. I was extremely nervous and full of disclaimers about being able to participate in our weekend together: I might not be able to go out with them, stay awake the full day, get dressed quickly, or cut and eat my dinner without their help. I would pull them back, I worried—and set off a flare-up amid all the stimulation and activity. How could they understand?

As it ended up, my friends and I turned my needs into a game by transforming a large batch of negatives into a collective, positive joke and painting a more intense picture that I hoped would help them comprehend my difficulties. Reminiscent of our summer camp days, we made a weekend "ElenOlympics" announcement for all participants, listing each need/difficulty as an activity assigned to one friend, with a contest embedded in the process: Whoever helped me cut my meat, turn a doorknob, comb my hair, fasten my bra, or reach over and properly "mooch" someone else's snacks (a tradition I was known for in this group) would win. The competition was on! And the pressure was off of me.

Simply walking through the process and listing my concerns with a friend helped to break down what had seemed to be an impenetrable barrier between my friends and me. When I talk of my next progress update for others, I have joked that I will send a portfolio of "what Elena's doing now," including a snapshot of myself just about to cut down a tree with an axe—or playing the piano to a full concert audience.

Look for ways in which you and your loved ones can do the same to gain perspective and entertain yourselves in tough times when you find yourself in inconceivable situations. Dark humor is not necessarily tactless. I daresay the darkest moments sometimes can only be illuminated by laughter.

Understanding Yourself

Adapting to caring for someone with CRPS is difficult for spouses, friends, and other family members, regardless of the severity of the condition. As much as your loved one needs your help, remember that being the best person you need to be for him or her includes taking steps to keep yourself "whole."

Taking Stock of Emotions

As much as you wish to care for your loved one in the best way possible, it's important to know early on that it is impossible to be a caregiver "gracefully" all the time. No book or guide can prevent you from passing through this experience as an emotional and psychological virgin to CRPS caregiving. No matter how strong a relationship, no matter how much effort you breathe into your service, and no matter how tough you think you are, the negative emotions hitting your loved one will also find their way to you. Let's take stock of a few of them.

You'll have your own anger: anger toward others who have overlooked or abandoned your loved one and/or you, anger at your helplessness in the situation, anger projected onto the sufferer ("If she really tried hard enough, she could beat this."), and finally anger toward yourself for feeling anger toward the sufferer.

You'll have your own grief. Certain dreams you had for yourself or together with your loved one are now on hold or possibly must be reworked, and you have lost many elements of your daily lifestyle and activities under these completely new rules of engagement. You have lost certain carefree parts of yourself and wrapped them up in another's concerns.

You'll have your own guilt: guilt for going out and enjoying something in the outside world and knowing that your loved one is in pain from not being able to experience it himself or herself; guilt for not doing enough for this person, while at the same time you know that you are barely doing enough for yourself.

You'll have your own fears. What is to become of your loved one as well as yourself? Will you be able to sustain both of you? Financially, professionally, emotionally and psychologically, you're under immense strain amid incredible chaos and uncertainty. You may fear that you're losing yourself. Will your health fail, too?

It's important to know that these feelings are normal and part of the process. Being constructively honest and open about these feelings—with yourself and with others—is the best way to manage them in the long-term. Most of all: *Do not feel bad for feeling bad.*

Nurturing Yourself

The person with CRPS may need help, but that doesn't preclude the fact that you need to have your own support network to lean on as well. Let others in. Let them read this chapter! Let them know what you're going through, so that you at least do not have to be the only link in understanding this condition.

I watched my mother become pathologically involved in my own well-being, and what happened provides a very clear example of the altruistic but potentially dehumanizing experience of intense caregiving. After moving over two thousand miles and returning home to live with her, I found my mother quickly became my guardian, my link to the outside world, and the only person who fully understood every ounce of my physical, emotional, and psychological distress. I realized how lucky I was to not feel completely alienated because I only had to sigh, and she knew what I was feeling. This connection was vital for me psychologically. However, I also watched my mother's health rapidly deteriorate as she further lost touch with others and became consumed with helping me get better. Rather than working as a stockbroker, she spent her time on housework, helping me with activities of daily living, errands, medication, doctor's appointments, and the piles and piles of paperwork that I could not fill out with my hands. Slowly, we were spiraling away onto our own "Planet RSD," as we called it at the time, and I watched it take its toll on my mother's own health and relationships.

Eventually, some balance was regained when I found myself in an improved physical condition, only to find myself stuck in an emotional and psychological trench that two people were then sharing. Without a doubt, my mother's unhappiness was affecting my unhappiness, and the only way to fix the situation for both of us was for her to reconnect with the things she loved again. She began nurturing herself, taking time to listen to her own voice, and actually started practicing many of the stress-relief and self-nourishing complementary practices that I had learned in my own pain-management efforts. She began using yoga tapes—and would not do them with me in the room; this was her private time, her session. She began dancing around to music she loved again, to awaken her energies and joy. She started working again, and her connection to the outside world at a job she loved was one of the best things she could have done for the next step in my own healing. The feeling of the "outside world" that she brought in with her was refreshing in the house. It was rejuvenating and gave us a feeling of connectedness, as if we were not all alone on our own planet anymore (even if that incubation period did have to occur originally).

Without a doubt, a caregiver is on a journey of finding a voice true to him- or herself while also being available for another. You have to be selfish sometimes. You have to take the time to participate in a hobby, have some fun, do your own thing, and separate yourself from this intense engagement with your loved one's pain. You have to take the time to examine how these moments of chaos impact you personally. And, in turn, there will be some common ways for you and your loved one to both nurture yourselves and share in an activity together—to form a new type of connection. Check Chapters 6 and 7 and the patient stories scattered throughout the book to review many practices and activities that can support and serve you as well as the person with CRPS.

Seeking Support

Friends and family members are a great place to start when seeking support. Try not to think about being a "burden" to others and don't hold back in fear of their judgment. This is what life is all about, but many people just have not come across this intensely transformative type of challenge yet.

Following are some of the many people to communicate with about your feelings and needs:

+ your local church, synagogue, or mosque
+ a psychologist or therapist
+ a support group for caregivers at a local hospital or pain clinic
+ national caregiver organizations, their support groups, and their chat rooms
+ CRPS/RSD and chronic pain associations

For a list of helpful organizations, please see the Resources section at the back of this book.

Celebrating and Affirming

Remember, being a caregiver can make *you* ill. It's most important to take care of yourself and remind yourself of the joys you are allowed upon waking up every morning. Your dreams, your joys, your silly thoughts, and your spirituality need to buoy you and keep you from sinking beneath the heavy burden of another's pains.

However miniscule the joy or advancement in healing, give yourself and your loved one the gift of marking and celebrating it. To remind yourself of your own full capacity and individual destiny, keep a copy of Sefra Kobrin Pitzele's *Kind Words for Caring People: Daily Affirmations for Caregivers* on your night table. It offers 365 inspiring, hopeful thoughts and ideas, allowing you to read a message every morning and reread it before going to sleep.

Everyone Can Get Involved: Working to Increase Awareness of CRPS

A recurrent theme in almost everyone's CRPS/RSD story—patient and doctor—is the painful maze sufferers had to wander through before obtaining a diagnosis. Many medical professionals are simply unaware of CRPS or never think to look for it; others disagree about what constitutes CRPS and even question fellow colleagues' diagnoses. Amid this internal confusion, the CRPS–RSD name changes can add an extra barrier to awareness. As if this were not distressing enough, awareness and understanding about the condition in the general population are low, especially compared to knowledge about other rare neurological conditions, such as multiple sclerosis (MS).

In a study conducted by a European CRPS website regarding the most crucial problem surrounding CRPS, respondents overwhelmingly emphasized the great need for increased awareness of the condition. Not only do patients highlight this challenge, but also doctors who are themselves CRPS patients tell of being mishandled, dismissed, or subjected to aggravating surgeries at the hands of their medical peers. One clinical psychologist, director of his department at a hospital, expressed his grief at being dismissed regarding the intensity of his pain. Another oncologist, claiming he did not know what CRPS was before he got it, claimed, "I put myself in the hands of colleagues I trusted then but that in the end turned out to be totally ignorant, inexperienced surgeons [who] advocated unnecessary, ill-advised, and technically poor surgeries (two of them). It is extremely hard to stay away from the feelings of anger and disrespect for the individuals [who] contributed to this situation, mainly due to their complete ignorance, arrogance, lack of understanding, and false, blind belief in their ability to fix problems through invasive, surgical means."

With increased awareness, the following objectives benefiting the CRPS population may finally be achieved:

◆ Making RSD/CRPS a known household condition would help the general population learn about how to approach, empathize with, and assist sufferers

◆ Providing warning information to patients about the possible development or exacerbation of CRPS before certain surgeries

◆ Making training and recertification programs mandatory for surgeons and orthopedists to prepare them for identifying RSD

◆ Offering preparatory training for doctors, nurses, physical therapists, dentists, and occupational therapists to help them become vigilant in recognizing early symptoms

◆ Training other medical professionals to prepare them for accommodating patients with CRPS and not exacerbating the patients' conditions

◆ Including uniform educational materials at medical websites to help patients understand what is happening in their bodies

Unfortunately, even within the expert community of researchers and doctors who treat CRPS extensively or publish articles on it, the controversy of what constitutes CRPS has jumped from professional to professional. Some doctors are discredited for "over-diagnosing" CRPS, some for "underdiagnosing" it, and others for performing treatments that can be harmful (e.g., radiofrequency or chemical sympathectomies). Where does that leave the average CRPS patient?

Rather than getting caught up in this higher level of controversy, breaking awareness efforts into smaller pieces might be just the method for fueling bigger and broader change. Here's how each of us can start.

Daily Communication

Imagine how many people come into contact with your snail mail or e-mail every day. Adding the website of your RSD/CRPS organization of choice at the bottom of your e-mails or at the top left-hand corner of an envelope is a simple method of increasing the odds of people coming into contact with it, and more people will be driven to look it up without you having to specifically mention or discuss it. Whether you include it in your automatic outbound e-mail signature, stationery, or preprinted return address labels, setting up a system for daily communication awareness can be cost-free, quick, and effective.

Pamphlet Distribution

Organizations such as the Reflex Sympathetic Dystrophy Syndrome Association of America (RSDSA) or RSD/CRPS United Kingdom have pamphlets available about RSD that you can order and distribute. Think of how many people might be reached if you and your loved ones picked just a few local grocery stores, churches, synagogues, health clubs, libraries, pharmacies, and your own doctors' offices and placed pamphlets there, alongside other community notices. Look around your neighborhood; you'll see there's always a medical fundraiser charity brochure in your midst. Follow this lead: Approach the shop owner in charge of pamphlet displays, and ask if you can leave out a few pamphlets of your own. Grassroots efforts like this can really make a difference!

For guidance on how you can make a difference—no matter how large or small—the For Grace foundation kicked off a National Awareness Campaign in October 2003. As a Web-based forum at http://forums.delphiforums.com/forgracenac/start, it provides a meeting place for you to share ideas and download specific tools and resources to increase awareness on a personal level. For example, handouts and business cards reviewing CRPS, posters that you can have printed out in larger sizes at a copy shop, sample press releases, guidance on public speaking, and other media aids and tips are included. RSDSA also provides a publicity kit on its website, including speech and news release ideas that you can customize for your local community newsletter or club.

Awareness Months and Days

Various organizations have established awareness months and days in order to focus awareness efforts for greatest visibility. If you're looking for a good time to increase your awareness efforts, consider launching them during an established awareness month. It is a great way to create momentum, as others around you will be doing the same. November is national RSD/CRPS awareness month in the United States and United Kingdom. Check CRPS/RSD association websites (listed in the Resources section) to keep up-to-date on their activities—or make a call to your local newspaper or community club to add to the buzz. Print and television media, bike races, bake sales, and walks will create visibility for the CRPS awareness efforts in progress.

Another option includes participating and offering your story for more local awareness during certain state-selective months or weeks. For example, Pennsylvania has just pushed through an awareness program, as has Illinois; November is RSD awareness month for Maine; and California has established May as RSD awareness month. The California bill was pushed through via a state senate hearing on the condition—the first of its kind—thanks to the efforts of For Grace. The passage of the bill made it obligatory for California policy makers to learn about this condition. If you're interested in participating in these local events or wish to try to push through your own state's awareness legislation, check the For Grace or RSDSA websites for sample letters and other materials necessary for working such a campaign.

You can also join forces with more general pain organizations, such as the American Pain Society, the Canadian Pain Society, and the British Pain Society. The American Pain Society, in conjunction with Partners Against Pain, has declared September to be National Pain Awareness Month; October features a European Week Against Pain.

Fund-Raising

Having a support network to advocate collectively on the behalf of CRPS patients is invaluable. Fundraising enables CRPS/RSD organizations to connect individuals to resources, medical advisors to educational campaigns, and dollars to research. Below are ways you can get involved in fueling these efforts.

Supplies

Nonprofit organizations working to raise awareness of CRPS need money for big campaigns as well as for the basics. Printing, envelopes, paper, pens, and stamps—even website support—are all critical to their success. You can help by supplying these necessities directly or raising the money to purchase them.

Merchandise

You can also assist by buying CRPS awareness merchandise. RSD/CRPS United Kingdom sells Christmas cards and calendars. Other organizations, such as the RSDS Association of America, offer badges and ribbons (much like the AIDS or breast-cancer ribbons) for sale. Imagine how many people would be curious and would ask about your RSD lapel badge—especially if they learned that a broken finger or stubbed toe could develop into this condition. Check the organizations listed in the Resources section and search their websites for available merchandise.

Online Retailers

The website www.igive.com offers you and others the chance to purchase items from 428 stores, including Spiegel, J. Crew, Avon, and other retailers while ensuring that the RSDS Association of America receives a donated percentage of the sale. When you visit the site, specify the association as your preferred charity and check to see what percentage each retailer will individually donate. Then pass along this information to all your e-mail buddies and colleagues!

Charitable Gift-Giving

Another option is gift giving. For example, if someone plans to give a present in honor of a birthday, ask if she or he can instead offer a donation in your name to the CRPS/RSD association of your choice. Employers may even participate in a matching gift program, which doubles the gift amount offered. Umbrella organizations, such as the United Way, include the RSDS Association of America as a Charity of Choice, and donors can specify this organization as the recipient. Finally, the RSDS Association of America is a member of Health and Medical Research Charities of America.

Letter Writing

Keep up-to-date on the latest legislation being advocated by your organization of choice. Whether it is the National Pain Care Policy Act or other campaigns being carried out at a higher level, see if you can add to the buzz by writing a letter to your elected representative. The RSDS Association of America and other pain-care organizations post their latest campaigns on their websites and offer downloads of sample letters you can date, print out, and send to your local congressperson.

Or how about writing a letter to the editor of your local paper that simply announces the existence of CRPS and your experience with it? Don't worry if you've never written a letter before or have never considered yourself a writer. It does not have to be a refined article; however, numerous readers will skim this part of the newspaper and come across something they might never have heard of before. Your human interest story is compelling. Consider including the address for a website to your CRPS association of choice, so readers can gather more information there. PARC (Promoting Awareness and Research in Canada) provides a preprepared editor's letter for members. It is a great sample to follow and customize.

Petitions

Keep up-to-date with CRPS and pain-related petitions calling for action, such as the one from Women Against Pain demanding a stop to gender bias in evaluating severity and seriousness of physical pain in women. The latest petitions are always posted prominently on association websites. Find them at places such as www .petitiononline.com/winpain/petition.html, sign them, and pass them on.

Informal Medical Professional Education

I read an inspiring letter about a couple who was slowly educating the medical professionals in their region about CRPS. This might seem impossible, but if your doctors seem receptive and willing to learn, a wonderful CRPS medical professional slide kit is available for them to see, courtesy of the RSDS Association of America.

The PowerPoint presentation can be found at www.rsds.org/3/edu cation. Every informed doctor counts. Who knows? Maybe these doctors will use this presentation to educate their colleagues. The RSDS Association of America also offers "Telltale signs of RSD/ CRPS type 1" handicards for free. You can distribute these at your physician's or therapist's office also.

It's also important to remember that a number of organizations such as PARC (Promoting Awareness and Research in Canada) and the RSDS Association of America do their own legwork by directly educating doctors. For example, PARC provides informational fact sheets on diagnosis and management of RSD and newsletters to the doctors of every CRPS patient who contacts them. RSDS Association of America organizes conferences and institutes for medical professionals and patients alike, including a Physical Therapist/Occupational Therapist Institute specifically instructing therapists on CRPS treatment protocols and methods.

Speakers Bureau

If you're a member of a community organization such as the Lions Club or a neighborhood church, it's a little-known fact that members of medical professional organizations, such as the American Osteopathic Association, have people available to speak to your group on an issue of your choice. As CRPS touches so many different professional disciplines, check the medical organizations in the Resources section and see if someone from one of these organizations might want to come out and educate your group.

Caregiver Awareness

Finally, CRPS deeply affects both caregivers and patients. November is National Family Caregivers Month. During this time, town hall meetings and other events offer a focused opportunity and news hook for caregivers to convey their needs. To find out how you can aid this year's efforts for these unsung heroes, call the National Family Caregivers Association at (800) 896-3650. Or write a letter to your local paper and share your story. Each person who reads it matters!

❖ ❖ ❖

Read Derrick's story to learn how one CRPS patient launched a website to increase public awareness of the condition. Derrick and a group of other volunteers operated an RSD awareness website for many years at a time when patients in the UK were first beginning to connect to others online.

errick's Story

When I set out to climb Dartmoor's two highest peaks one bright January day in 1999, I didn't expect it to be a life-changing experience. Neither mountain peak was visible when I began my walk, as the overnight mist was still hugging the slopes, waiting for the sun to burn it off. The air was cold but still, and clear pools of ice lay where water had seeped into the gaps among the rocks.

After a brief lunch I set out across the pass to the lesser-known but higher peak to enjoy the clear view from the top, before heading back to the car and home. The return path was well laid and almost level, so I strolled along happy and unhurried. Then I stepped on a rock that still had a covering of frost. My fall was so sudden that I have no memory of the instant before I found myself, dazed and startled, on the ground. Falling in such a safe and level place, I felt stupid but not hurt. It seemed like a trivial accident until I realized that I had no control over my left hand. [My arm] was obviously broken.

Mine was the fifth broken arm they had seen that day at the hospital, as the frost that caught me had also turned Plymouth's streets into ice rinks. My accident was one among many and, for all the expected inconvenience, still only a broken arm. But, as the weeks wore on, my pain persisted and got worse. Eventually, my arm swelled so much that the plaster had to be slit to relieve the pressure. When the cast came off, it revealed a pitifully stiff and crooked hand and the first angry signs of CRPS [which was called RSD at the time].

I had never heard of reflex sympathetic dystrophy, so the significance of the diagnosis did not strike me until one of my sons surfed the Internet for information and phoned me in some concern. When I looked it up myself, I saw what he meant. There was not much about RSD on the Internet, but what there was made it seem pretty horrific. A number of sufferers told stories about terrible, increasing pain, and hardly any held out hope for recovery or relief.

Eventually, I found a hint that remission might be possible for people who were diagnosed early, if they worked hard at physical therapy. It sounded like a wake-up call, and I took it very seriously. Never have I willingly accepted so much pain. For nine months I underwent weekly sessions with the physiotherapist and worked hard at the exercises four times a day—and it hurt! But gradually, I began to win small triumphs, like touching my thumb to my fingers, tearing a tissue off a roll, buttoning a shirt, or lacing a shoe. Eventually, I was able to drive my car again and even play my guitar.

The Internet had contributed to my deliverance, and I wanted to give something back. However, I wanted to make it positive, to raise hope, to encourage people rather than frighten them, and I wanted to deliver facts. The Internet was still in its early days—quickly becoming newsworthy, but still a year away from its explosion into everyday culture for the millions. But I figured that my small story and its positive outcome would be able to help at least a few people. So I published the story on one of my own websites. It was a personal testimony and only a few pages long, but it soon became evident that many people were finding and appreciating it.

I guess that many volunteers are like me; you take something on and gradually find that it is bigger than you realized when you started. Don't believe anyone who tells you that RSD is rare. It is much more common than many well-publicized medical conditions, but when I first posted my story on the Internet, most people had never heard of it because few people were championing the cause. The more successful my website became, the more I got sucked into running it. Then I needed people to help, and volunteers came forward. Gradually we made contact with other groups and websites and started cooperating to increase our effectiveness. Eventually we had as many visitors each day as found the site in our first year. Thousands of people found information, help, and encouragement, and a portion of them achieved remission.

The word *remission* has the ominous sound of a threat that still hangs over your head, which *is* the reality of CRPS. My hand and wrist have been free of pain for over four years—but I cannot guarantee that [they] will stay that way. CRPS still lurks in the background, giving me strange sensations in my wrist—but not pain. What I can guarantee is that if the condition flares up again, it will find me ready to fight back. I have never stopped doing the exercises to keep my joints supple and active, and I won't stop the battle to make the world aware of complex regional pain syndrome. My Sunday morning walk turned into a lifelong awareness campaign.

Getting Started

You may feel as if you want to help, but you're overwhelmed or do not know where to start. Bear in mind that you do not have to start your own nonprofit organization, launch your own website, or spend numerous hours doing volunteer work to make a difference. Every little action makes a difference. Please check the Resources section for websites and/or contact information of CRPS and pain organizations to begin participating in an initiative or two.

The more awareness people have about CRPS, the easier it will be for patients to obtain an accurate diagnosis and crucial, speedy treatment—and receive the support they need in the rest of their lives as well. The more we all know, the more we can advance. You've already come this far; take your first step on this new advocacy path today!

A Parting Perspective

What a trek this has been. It has proven more difficult than I ever expected to write this book and at the same time to remain true to myself and to you, the reader. Let me explain what I mean.

As it happens, I find myself completing this project when I am healthier than I was before. One of the greatest defenses our brains offer us against severe pain is a faded memory. On a daily basis, I lock behind the doors to my subconscious the deepest, most horrifying fears, despair, and sensations I felt at the onset of my CRPS. To make room for progress, I willed myself to dismiss trauma as soon as it loosened its grip on me. To be true to this book, however, I had to unlock those doors and once again explore those moments. The keys to the doors were the hundreds of patients' stories I received that detailed their struggles and the dozens of research articles I read that addressed specific clinical symptoms I had also endured.

Once I began delving into my past experiences with CRPS, I was surprised by how much I had forgotten of my early excruciating moments. It seemed I'd put them behind me as easily as I'd forgotten the "sick clothes" now banished from my wardrobe (I threw them out because they contained such negative energy for me). Yet refocusing my memory on those times, those symptoms, and all the confusion that had swirled around in my head made my heart beat fast, my breath come short, my stomach swell with nausea, and a cry well up in the back of my throat.

A decade later, in this updated book edition, I'm again unpacking pieces of the experience that were too traumatic to ruminate on at the time—yet inform who I am today—and the fears I quietly manage with regards to relapse. I want you to know that I and other individuals are thinking about your struggles and your pains every day. Know that you're not alone in your efforts with CRPS; people out there understand the depth of your challenges. That is the primary message I want you to take away from this book. Take too that meaningful change is possible in many cases—even if it takes years to get there.

Here's something else to remember as you take in all the information contained in this book: Break it down and digest it in small pieces. The questions about what will happen with your relationships, your kids, your financial situation, the career you worked hard for, the next doctor you'll see, the test results, when you will walk again, when you can sign your name or open a jar again, when you will sleep soundly all night, when or if the nerve block will wear off, how much the medications will cost, what will happen to you, and how you will be feeling in the next hour, the next day, for the next five years, for the rest of your life—these are all too large to get your head around and solve at once! Take it one issue at a time, and remember that these questions can never be answered with certainty, even by "normal" healthy folks. Because I'm a multitasker and an overanalyzer, surrendering all of these "what ifs" has been an ongoing process for me. Yet shutting off the tendency to let my entire life flash before my eyes when I face a setback has helped me enormously. Please, give it a try.

Managing CRPS requires tightrope walking. How else can you embrace "healing" in lieu of a "cure"? How else can you walk the precarious line between hope and acceptance? Even those of us in remission would like to imagine that we've completely excised the

CRPS demon. It's important to know that just because you might have to continue managing this chronic condition, loss and fear don't have to hijack your visions of the future. Create a safe space in your psyche to accommodate these uncertainties and gray spots. Nurture yourself every day. Mark this time in your life as a period of deep transformation. Learning to live well with CRPS is another ongoing process.

It's interesting to contemplate how the many and varied healing paths adopted by CRPS patients can differ so widely. Using a variety of mental tools, I tapped into the power of my inner creative spirit to help me through moment-to-moment challenges. By contrast, many others find their strength in religious practice. Elizabeth, now age fifty-five, developed CRPS following carpal tunnel surgery in December 1994. In her story she shares how important it is to find skilled and caring practitioners, talks about the usefulness of utilizing what she calls "memory tactics," and describes how she learned to hear and follow her inner guidance, a skill that proved crucial to managing her health. She also talks about taking sanctuary in her dialogues with God.

Elizabeth's Story

I went in for a "simple" surgery by a top-notch doctor at a wonderful hospital. Post-op, I met CRPS and all its horrendous pain. It made a quick assault on my upper extremities—as well as on my resilient spirit! Unlike many others, I was diagnosed correctly and immediately. I welcomed all the conventional wisdom and help offered by my terrific medical team. I consulted with hand therapists, physical therapists, and ultimately with practitioners of alternative health methods, including acupuncture, massage therapy, nutritional guidance, and water therapy. I learned all I could about CRPS.

I have always considered myself a problem solver who looked for the best in people and situations. I was respected for my personal integrity, leadership skills, and positive outlook. I enjoyed fixing a bad situation and helping people. After I was diagnosed with CRPS, when I was confronted with the loss of my hard-earned career, I hit bottom.

When I realized the consequences of my pain on our home life and on my treasured independence, I knew I had to shift, or CRPS would become a new boss. I remember my husband said that I should drop the worries about my job loss and focus on what would be the most challenging job of my life: healing me. Focusing on myself was new.

As I turned my attention to my new number-one problem, I was thankful for the team of experts I was able to put together. Once I felt "safe" in their care, I was able to approach my healing process with conviction and hope. In time, I learned what personality traits served me well and what did not. Coping with a suicidal level of pain became both a physical and emotional challenge. I quickly recognized the value of those who supported me and not only refrained from judging my decisions but also honored them. The professionals I was fortunate enough to have engaged in my care gave me this precious gift.

Over time, I came to value my amazing body and all of its complexities. I listened to it and felt every level of pain reaction. All the circuitry of energy became clearer to me. My challenge was to find ways to minimize assaults on my central nervous system. I reminded my brain-driven CRPS that it wasn't going to destroy any more of me, and I kept telling my arms not to lose function. I continued to remind my brain that I wanted it to return normalcy to my upper extremities. I call these "memory tactics." All the while, my deep faith and personal dialogue with God gave me strength and sanctuary. I was learning how to protect myself. Keeping calm is crucial to any level of healing. There is a vicious cycle of destructive tension that comes with acute and chronic pain. Finding calm in the center of that storm is critical.

We all can identify with anger and fear. I experienced the deep grieving process that goes along with catastrophic events. I learned all I could from a remarkable neurologist and her team. I was comforted by the healing hands of massage therapists and acupuncturists. They did and still do give me so much. I'm wiser because of them. I treasure the everyday moments more and try to override the chatter of the "what ifs." The anger is gone. I have good days and bad days, but the good outweigh the bad. I try to honor my ongoing maintenance program now by following my own inner direction. I have less pain, and I can see and feel improvement. I find it toxic to dwell upon CRPS!

Instead, I choose to measure myself by my more powerful traits and beliefs.

I know there is always some place in my body that doesn't have pain, and I seek it out. I'm very proud of my endeavors! I have grown personally, and I continue to hear my own spirit guide me. Instead of focusing on loss, I focus on gain. I understand the need to balance both my parasympathetic and sympathetic nervous systems, and when one is dwarfed by the other, I take note and find ways to channel balancing results. My internal "meter-reader" helps me.

Along the way, I found that my creative spirit wanted to be expressed in a different medium. I "travel" with a watercolor brush. I have discovered many levels of art expression, and it's been revealing, rewarding, calming, and healing. I have also learned that I can paint in my mind. If painting on paper is uncomfortable on a particular day, I can still embark into my imagination or collect ideas to execute later.

I respect the gift of life with deep reverence. I can honestly say CRPS has given me an opportunity to understand myself more than any other life experience. Of course, I wish the CRPS chapter of my life had never happened. However, I have gained deep insight about so much, and my problem-solving skills have proven to be a viable part of me!

I encourage anyone with chronic CRPS to treasure yourself and to forgive yourself when you neglect certain practices that help. Because I want to embrace life, I sometimes overdo it, and when that happens it's difficult to cope with the consequences. Still, I choose to try again.

It's clear that everyone will experience some painful or difficult experience during her lifetime. If we are able to rise above it, we can learn a level of internal peace that becomes a compass for other hard times. Look for inspiration, and at the same time be your own inspiration!

Change is an essential feature of CRPS. No one escapes this illness unscathed by some form of transformation. Your bodily functions, thought processes, worries, and self-image will all be tinged by CRPS. Think of these changes not as a stain on your former life but as a new chapter. Parts of yourself that perhaps lay dormant and abilities that previously remained untapped may now have to come to the forefront, like overlooked cast members who must take the lead role in a play. You might come across different value systems that work better for you at this point in your life. Flirt with them, learn from them, and seize them if you find them effective.

Don't waste time torturing yourself by thinking about how much easier things would be if you could just do them the "normal way"; find your baseline every day, and work from there. Most important, believe in yourself, believe in your capacity to change — and hold faith in your ability to endure, survive, and adapt.

References

Chapter 1: "What Is CRPS?"

Barad, M. J., T. Ueno, J. Younger, N. Chatterjee, and S. Mackey. 2014. Complex regional pain syndrome is associated with structural abnormalities in pain-related regions of the human brain. *Journal of Pain* 15, no. 2: 197–203. http://www.ncbi.nlm.nih.gov/pubmed/24212070 (accessed May 14, 2014).

Beerthuizen, A., D. Stronks, A. Van't Spijker, A. Yaksh, B. Hanraets, J. Klein, and F. Huygen. 2012. Demographic and medical parameters in the development of complex regional pain syndrome type 1 (CRPS1): Prospective study on 596 patients with a fracture. *Pain* 153:1187–92.

Bruehl, S. 2010. An update on the pathophysiology of complex regional pain syndrome. *Anesthesiology* 113:713–25.

Carden, E. 2002. Reflex sympathetic dystrophy: Recognition and management for the physician. Paper, Southern California Academic Pain Management, Santa Monica.

Cooper, M., and V. Clark. 2012. Neuroinflammation, neuroautoimmunity, and the co-morbidities of complex regional pain syndrome. *Journal of Neuroimmune Pharmacology* 8, no. 3: 452–69. http://link.springer.com/article/10.1007%2Fs11481-012-9392-x (accessed May 14, 2014).

Finding an RSD specialist. 1999. *RSDSA News*, 1–4.

Finding Help for Your Pain. 2002. Publication of American Pain Foundation.

Hendler, N. 1995. Reflex sympathetic dystrophy: Clearing up the misconceptions. *The Journal of Workers' Compensation* 5: 9–19.

Livingstone, W. 1943. *Pain mechanisms: A physiological interpretation of causalgia and its related states.* London: McMillan.

Maihofner, C., F. Seifert, and K. Markovic. 2010. Complex regional pain syndromes: New pathophysiological concepts and therapies. *European Journal of Neurology* 17, no. 5: 649–60.

Maihofner, C., H. O. Handwerker, B. Neundörfer, and F. Birklein. 2003. Patterns of cortical reorganization in complex regional pain syndrome. *Neurology* 61:1707–1715.

National Institutes of Health. 2004. *Reflex sympathetic dystrophy.* Fact sheet from U.S. Department of Health and Human Services, National Institutes of Health, Bethesda, MD.

Reflex Sympathetic Dystrophy Syndrome Association. 2000. *Clinical practice guidelines.* Ed. A.F. Kirkpatrick, published by Reflex Sympathetic Dystrophy Association.

Reuben, S., E. A. Rosenthal, R. B. Steinberg, S. Faruqi, and P. A. Kilaru. 2004. Surgery on the affected upper extremity of patients with a history of complex regional pain syndrome: The use of intravenous regional anesthesia with clonodine. *Journal of Clinical Anesthesia* 16: 517–22.

Schwartzman, R. 2012. Systemic complications of complex regional pain syndrome. *Neuroscience and Medicine.* http://www.scirp.org /journal/nm (accessed January 3, 2014).

Schwenkreis, P., F. Janssen, and O. Rommel. 2003. Bilateral motor cortex disinhibition in complex regional pain syndrome (CRPS) type 1 of the hand. *Neurology* 61:515–19.

Sheon, R. P. 2003. Reflex sympathetic dystrophy (complex regional pain syndrome) in adults. Website: UptoDate, version 11.3. Online literature review through September 2003. www.utdol.com (accessed July 5, 2003).

Shirani, P., A. Jawaid, P. Moretti, E. Lahijani, A. Salamone, P. Schulz, and E. Edmondson. 2010. Familial occurrence of complex regional pain syndrome. *Canadian Journal of Neurological Science* 37: 389–94.

Vacariu, G. 2002. Complex regional pain syndrome. *Disability and Rehabilitation* 24:435–42.

Wasner, G., J. Schattschneider, A. Binder, and R. Baron. 2003. Complex regional pain syndrome: diagnostics, mechanisms, CNS involvement, and therapy. *Spinal Cord* 41: 61–75.

Zollinger, P. E., W. E. Tuinebreijer, R. W. Kreis, and R. S. Breederveld. 1999. Effect of vitamin C on frequency of reflex sympathetic dystrophy in wrist fractures: A randomized trial. *Lancet* 354, no. 9195: 2025–28.

Chapter 2: "Treatment Options for CRPS"

Biofeedback FAQ: Getting started as a professional. www.futurehealth .org (accessed February 5, 2004).

Carden, E. 2002. Reflex sympathetic dystrophy: Recognition and management for the physician. Paper, Southern California Academic Pain Management, Santa Monica.

Correll, G. E., J. Maleki, E. J. Gracely, J. J. Muir, and R. E. Harbut. 2004. Subanesthetic ketamine infusion therapy: A retrospective analysis of a novel therapeutic approach to complex regional pain syndrome. *Pain Medicine* 5, no. 3: 263–75.

Ek, J. W., J. van Gijn, H. Samuel, J. van Egmond, F. Klomp, and R. van Dongen. 2009. Pain exposure physical therapy may be a safe and effective treatment for long-standing complex regional pain syndrome type I: A case series. *Clinical Rehabilitation* 23:1059–66.

Fonoff, E. T., C. Hamani, D. Ciampi de Andrade, L. T. Yeng, M. A. Marcolin, and M. J. Teixeira. 2011. Pain relief and functional recovery in patients with complex regional pain syndrome after motor cortex stimulation. *Stereotactic and Functional Neurosurgery* 89: 167–72.

Hendler, N. 1995. Reflex sympathetic dystrophy: Clearing up the misconceptions. *The Journal of Workers' Compensation* 5: 9–19.

Kiefer, R. T., P. Rohr, A. Ploppa, H. J. Dieterich, J. Grothusen, S. Koffler, K. H. Altemeyer, K. Unertl, and R. J. Schwartzman. 2008. Efficacy of ketamine and anesthetic dosage for the treatment of refractory complex regional pain syndrome: an open-label phase 2 study. *Pain Medicine* 9, no. 8: 1173–201.

Lang, L., and P. Moskovitz. 2003. *Living with RSDS*. Oakland CA: New Harbinger.

Lee, S. K., D. S. Yang, J. W. Lee, and W. S. Choy. 2012. Four treatment strategies for complex regional pain syndrome type I. *Orthopedics* 35:e834–42.

Maihöfner, C., F. Seifert, and K. Markovic. 2010. Complex regional pain syndromes: New pathophysiological concepts and therapies. *European Journal of Neurology* 17, no. 5: 649–60.

Marineo, G., G. Iorno, C. Gandini, V. Moschini, and T. Smith. 2012. Scrambler therapy may relieve chronic neuropathic pain more effectively than guideline-based drug management: Results of a pilot, randomized, controlled trial. *Journal of Pain and Symptom Management* 43: 87–95.

Perez, R. 2002. CRPS 1: A randomized controlled study into the effects of two free-radical scavengers and evaluation of measurement instruments. Thesis. ISBN no. 90-9015456-6.

Raja, S. N. 2002. Complex regional pain syndrome one (RSD) guidelines for therapy: Research outcomes versus expert opinions. Paper presented at the international update on RSD/CRPS. Tampa, FL.

Reflex Sympathetic Dystrophy Syndrome Association. 2000. *Clinical practice guidelines.* Ed. A. F. Kirkpatrick.

Schwartzman, R., et al. 2003. Is high-dose ketamine a therapeutic option for severe intractable complex regional pain syndrome type 1? American Society of Anesthesiologists Abstract. Meeting, San Francisco, CA.

Sigtermans, M. J., J. J. van Hilten, M. C. Bauer, M. S. Arbous, J. Marinus, E. Y. Sarton, and A. Dahan. 2009. Ketamine produces defective and long-term pain relief in patients with complex regional pain syndrome type 1. *Pain* 145, no. 3:304–311. http://www.ncbi.nlm.nih .gov/pubmed/19604642 (accessed April 11, 2014).

Stanton-Hicks, M., R. Baron, R. Boas, T. Gordh, N. Harden, N. Hendler, M. Koltzenburg, P. Raj, and R. Wilder. 1998. Complex regional pain syndromes: Guidelines for therapy. *The Clinical Journal of Pain* 14:155–64.

Stanton-Hicks, M. 2010. Plasticity of complex regional pain syndrome (CRPS) in children. *Pain Medicine* 11, no. 8:1216–23.

Vacariu, G. 2002. Complex regional pain syndrome. *Disability and Rehabilitation* 24:435–42.

Van der Laan, G. 2001. Reflex sympathetic dystrophy: Another view. *European Journal of Trauma* 27:99–103.

Van Eijs, F., M. Stanton-Hicks, J. Van Zundert, C. Faber, T. Lubenow, N. Mekhail, M. van Kleef, and F. Huygen. 2011. Evidence-based interventional pain medicine according to clinical diagnoses: Complex regional pain syndrome. *Pain Practice* 11:70–87.

Chapter 6: "A World of Support: Complementary Therapies"

Benson, H. 1984. *Beyond the Relaxation Response.* New York: Time Books. 1–18; 68–71.

DeSalvo, L. 1999. *Writing as a way of healing: How telling our stories transforms our lives.* San Francisco: HarperCollins.

Devi, S. 2002. *Yoga and pain: Finding peace of mind.* Publication of American Pain Foundation.

Gainer, M. J. 1992. Hypnotherapy for reflex sympathetic dystrophy. *American Journal of Clinical Hypnosis* 34: 227.

Goldberg, B. 2001. *Self-hypnosis.* Franklin Lakes, NJ: New Page Books. 1–25.

Hagedorn, R. 2001. *Foundations for practice in occupational therapy,* 3d ed. New York: Churchill Livingstone.

Hendler, N. 1984. Depression caused by chronic pain. *Journal of Clinical Psychiatry* 45:30–36.

Hinds, E. 2003. *A life larger than pain: The pathway from resignation to renewal.* Albuquerque, NM: Health Press.

Iyengar, B. K. S. 2001. *Yoga: The path to holistic health.* London: Dorling Kindersley.

Maihöfner, C., F. Seifert, and K. Markovic. 2010. Complex regional pain syndromes: New pathophysiological concepts and therapies. *European Journal of Neurology* 17, no. 5: 649–60.

Malchiodi, C. 1998. *The art therapy sourcebook.* Los Angeles: Lowell House.

Rama, S., R. Ballentine, and A Hymes. 1998. *Science of breath: A practical guide.* Honesdale, PA: The Himalayan Institute Press.

Sparadeo, F., C. Kaufman, and S. Amato. 2012. Scrambler therapy: An innovative and effective treatment for chronic neuropathic pain. *Journal of Life Care Planning* 11.

Varenna, M., S. Adami, M. Rossini, D. Gatti, L. Idolazzi, F. Zucchi, N. Malavolta, and L. Sinigaglia. 2013. Treatment of complex regional pain syndrome type I with neridronate: A randomized, double-blind, placebo-controlled study. *Rheumatology (Oxford)* 52: 534–42.

Walker, M. J., and J. Walker. 2003. *Healing massage: A simple approach.* Clifton Park, NY: Thomson Delmar Learning. 63–64; 80–100.

Weil, A. 1998. *Natural health, natural medicine.* Boston: Houghton Mifflin. 118–20.

Chapter 8: " Help for the Helper: A Chapter for Caregivers"

Wall, P. D., and R. Melzack. 1994. *Textbook of pain.* New York: Churchill Livingstone. 339–45.

Resources:
Where to Go from Here

You've read about your options in the previous chapters. Now here's the chance to act on them! I know how hard it is to know where to start, so I offer you a launching ground for your next steps, which may be in any direction you decide to pursue.

Research Studies and Experimental Treatments

The word *research* lights me up inside whenever I hear it in reference to CRPS. Any efforts to document patient cases, symptoms, probabilities, risks, and responses to certain treatments remind us of the possibilities out there—and we all have a part in shaping those possibilities. It's wise to consider the pros and cons of participating in a study that may help many, many people—including you!

At the time of updating this edition, several studies aim to increase understanding of CRPS pain and treatment. Basic details about a few of them are listed below. You can also keep current and find more information, such as exclusion criteria, by visiting the central http://clini caltrials.gov/ or other websites that post opportunities for patients to participate in clinical trials.

McGill University Research Projects
Qualifying patients are invited to participate in any one study or any combination of studies currently ongoing under the direction of Gary J. Bennett, PhD, whose past twenty-five years of research has focused on the mechanisms behind pain sensations. He is considered a pioneer of the theory that pain itself is a physiological abnormality. Studies last between one and a half and three hours, depending on the procedure. Stimuli are chosen to produce as little pain as possible. The studies include:

1. *Sensory testing for characterizing the details of the abnormal pain of RSD:* These studies apply precisely controlled touch, heat, and cold stimuli to the painful area and to normal areas to measure such things as the threshold for pain, the duration of the pain, the location of the pain, and so on.

2. *Functional magnetic resonance imaging (fMRI) studies:* MRI scans are taken while various stimuli (touch, cold, heat) are applied to the area of RSD and to normal areas.

3. *Scanning laser Doppler imaging of sympathetic nervous system reflexes:* This safe and noninvasive procedure consists of testing patients' responses to various stimuli, such as deep breathing maneuvers, while lightly brushing their skin.

4. *Skin biopsies:* Small, circular pieces of skin, three millimeters in diameter, are removed for chemical and anatomical study. The skin samples are taken after the skin is anesthetized. Researchers take two skin samples, one from painful skin and one from normal skin. (Researchers include the following note: "We realize that patients may be reluctant to participate in such an invasive study and we certainly respect anyone's decision not to participate. Although there is something obviously wrong with RSD skin, no one has ever examined it under the microscope to try to find exactly what is wrong.")

Patients receive a full medical evaluation from the physicians at the Montreal General Hospital Pain Centre.

Contact:
Gary J. Bennett, PhD
Anesthesia Research Unit
McGill University (McIntyre 1202)
Montreal, Quebec H3G 1Y6
Canada
(514) 398-3432
fax: (514) 398-8241
E-mail: gary.bennett@mcgill.ca

Botox for RSD/CRPS Patients

Patients with RSD/CRPS may be eligible to participate in a clinical research study conducted by the North Shore-LIJ Health System at the Cohn Pain Management Center.

Inclusion criteria:
- Subject must be eighteen to sixty-five years old.
- Subject must have complex regional pain syndrome type 1 (CRPS type 1)/RSD affecting one upper extremity only.
- Subject must be willing to undergo physical therapy treatments.
- Subject must have never received botox therapy for any reason.
- Subject must have not been treated with trigger point injections within the past month.

Contact:
Dr. Charles Argoff, Neurologist, or Margaret Rossi, Study Coordinator
Cohn Pain Management Center
4300 Hempstead Tpke.
Bethpage NY 11714
(516) 802-8673

Treatment of Complex Regional Pain Syndrome with Once Daily Gastric-Retentive Gabapentin (Gralise)

The study investigates the efficacy of gabapentin for the treatment of pain in CRPS I patients. Patients will be given the medication more than eight weeks, during which the functional benefits of the drug will recorded, with particular attention to the occurrence of side effects like dizziness, drowsiness, headaches, and swelling in the extremities that are known to occur when gabapentin is used to treat other conditions (neuralgia from shingles).

Inclusion Criteria:
- Subject will be 18 to 80 years of age.
- Subject has not been on Gralise.
- Subject has not been on gabapentin for at least one month.
- Subject agrees to make no change in his/her current pain medications during the study period to ensure that comparisons can be made before and after the Gralise treatment.
- Subject has a VAS pain score of 5 or above at the beginning of the study.
- Subject has had CRPS 1 for at least three months to avoid clinical uncertainty and minimize the study variation.

Contact:
Trang T. Vo, BA
Massachusetts General Hospital
Boston MA 02114
(617) 724-6102
tvo3@partners.org
Principal Investigator: Jianren Mao, MD, PhD

Investigation of the Efficacy of tDCS in the Treatment of Complex Regional Pain Syndrome (CRPS) Type 1

The study investigates a new nonpharmacological treatment for patients with CRPS 1 that applies electrical stimulation to the brain in order to reduce pain. This procedure, called transcranial direct current stimulation (tDCS), has shown promise when used to treat neuropathic pain in other studies, suggesting it may prove effective as an additional treatment method for CRPS I. This technology stimulates the affected area of the patient's motor cortex in order to inhibit pain in the affected limb. Patients participating in the study will be placed in two groups: One group will receive tDCS while the other receives a placebo treatment. Both groups will receive graded motor imagery (GMI) using well-established procedures, with the tDCS group receiving consecutive tDCS for five days during the first two weeks of the study. This constitutes the first phase of the study. The next two phases, lasting for four more weeks, will include tDCS administration once a week. The researchers hope to gather MRI/fMRI evidence documenting the structural changes that occur in the patient's brain as a result of the treatment and thereby shed light on the mechanism by which this technology may result in pain inhibition.

Inclusion Criteria:
- Adults (eighteen years and older) diagnosed with CRPS type 1, based on Bruehl's diagnostic criteria for research.

Contact:
Emilie Lagueux, OT PhD(c)
Université de Sherbrooke
Sherbrooke, Quebec
QC J1K 2R1 Canada
(819) 346-1110, ext 12436

emilie.lagueux@usherbrooke.ca
Principal Investigator: Yannick Tousignant-Laflamme, PhD

A Safety and Effectiveness Trial of Spinal Cord Stimulation of the Dorsal Root Ganglion for Chronic Lower Limb Pain

The study will be testing the safety and effectiveness of spinal cord stimulation for treating chronic lower limb pain in patients with CRPS or peripheral causalgia (PC). This trial will utilize a neurostimulator device designed to stimulate the dorsal root ganglion of the spinal cord in order to reduce pain. The device, called the AXIUM stimulator, will be surgically implanted in two parts: 1) a pulse generator that is placed under the skin in the buttocks or abdomen, and 2) up to four wires (leads) that have one end attached to the pulse generator and the other end secured to the tissue near the target treatment area. Control subjects will be implanted with a different stimulator device that is commercially available.

Inclusion Criteria:

- Subject is male or female between the ages of twenty-two and seventy-five years.
- Subject is able and willing to comply with the follow-up schedule and protocol.
- Subject has chronic, intractable pain of the lower limb(s) for at least six months.
- Subject is diagnosed with complex regional pain syndrome (CRPS) and/or peripheral causalgia.
- Subject has a minimum Visual Analog Scale for Pain (VAS) greater than or equal to 60 mm in the area of greatest pain in the lower limbs.
- Subject has failed to achieve adequate pain relief from at least two prior pharmacologic treatments from at least two different drugs classes.
- Subject has had stable neurologic function in the past thirty days.
- Subject, in the investigator's opinion, is psychologically appropriate for the implantation of an active implantable medical device.
- Subject is able to provide written informed consent.

Contact Information:
Linda Johnson, PhD
(650) 543-6800
linda@spinalmodulation.com

Steve McQuillan
(650) 543-6800
smcquillan@spinalmodulation.com

Sponsors and Collaborators: Spinal Modulation, Inc.
Study Locations: Throughout the United States.

Evaluation and Diagnosis of People with Pain and Fatigue Syndromes

The study examines people with pain syndromes in order to recruit appropriate candidates for the National Institute of Nursing Research (NINR) clinical trials pertaining to treatments for their condition. Participants will be screened using medical history information, physical examinations, routine laboratory tests, and questionnaires. These tests are designed to evaluate the candidate's level of pain and quality of life so that they can be matched to research studies that investigate treatments addressing their particular concerns. Patients who are found to be ineligible for NINR studies will be informed of alternative treatments. This study does not itself offer any treatments. Patients will only be directed to other protocols that may be beneficial to them.

Inclusion Criteria:
- Subject is eighteen years of age or older.
- Subject has symptoms of pain and/or fatigue.

Contact:
Leorey N. Saligan, CRNP
(301) 451-1685
saliganl@mail.nih.gov

Clinical Trial Websites
Canadian clinical trials
http://www.hc-sc.gc.ca/dhp-mps/prodpharma/databasdonclin/index
-eng.php

Clinical trials, U.S. and International
http://clinicaltrials.gov

Informed consent resources for patients
www.ecri.org/documents/clinical_trials_patient_reference_guide.pdf
www.amazon.com/Informed-Consent-Consumers-Benefits-Volunteer
ing/dp/1930624093

International clinical trial listing
www.centerwatch.com/cwworld/cwworld.html

Ongoing CRPS-pertinent study watch
www.rsdhope.org   www.rsds.org

Adaptive Equipment

Adaptive equipment includes kitchen accessories, walkers, walker accessories, canes, wheelchair accessories, magnets, exercise videos, gel cushions, gel mattresses, bathing and dressing aids, joint supports, splints, wraps, adapted utensils, reachers, bathroom safety equipment, and special products for caregivers. These websites can give you some ideas of what products are available. Additional recommendations gathered by patients on the Internet can be found at:

www.rsdcanada.org/parc/english/therapy/survival.html#9
www.thewright-stuff.com
www.pattersonmedical.com
www.ncmedical.com
www.independentliving.com
www.hdis.com/mobility.html
www.infinitec.org/live/kitchens/catalogsaids.htm

Scooters, Kneewalkers, and Wheelchairs
Scooter Link
www.scooterlink.com

Silver Cross
www.silvercross.com

Active Forever
www.activeforever.com/knee-walkers-scooters

Adaptive Driving
www.adaptivedriving.com

Caregiver Organizations
Caregivers Support Resources
The CAPP Caregiver Resource Center
The Mount Sinai Hospital
1 Gustave Levy Pl.
Box 1252
New York NY 10029
(212) 241-2277

Caregiver Action Network
2000 M St. NW, Ste. 400
Washington DC 20036
(202) 772-5050
http://caregiveraction.org
Provides resources, education, and support to family caregivers nationwide.

Caregivers Service
Health Outreach Office
New York Presbyterian Hospital
525 East 68th St., Box 143
New York NY 10131
(212) 746-4320

Family Caregiver Alliance
785 Market St., Ste. 750
San Francisco CA 94103
(800) 445-8106
(415) 434-3388
www.caregiver.org
Provides advocacy, training, education, and many other resources. For
family and friends providing long-term care at home.

The Family Caregiver Program
Beth Israel Medical Center
Department of Pain Medicine and Palliative Care
First Ave. at 16th St.
New York NY 10003
findhelp@netofcare.org
www.netofcare.org

Friend's Health Connection
P.O. Box 114
New Brunswick NJ 08903
(800) 48-FRIEND (483-7436)
(732) 418-1811
www.48friend.org
Connects caregivers with mutual support.

National Alliance for Caregiving
4720 Montgomery Ln., 2nd Fl.
Bethesda MD 20814-3425
(301) 718-8444
www.caregiving.org
Supports both caregivers and medical professionals who deal with caregivers, develops employed caregiver support and training programs, works on legislation, and offers other resources.

Rosalynn Carter Institute of Georgia Southwestern College
800 GSW Dr.
Americus GA 31709
(229) 928-1234
www.rci.gsw.edu
Hosts training programs for professionals and caregivers.

Caregiver Resource Centers Hosted by Hospitals
Well Spouse Foundation
63 West Main St.—Ste. H
Freehold NJ 07728
(800) 838-0879
www.wellspouse.org
Provides support to spouses/partners of the ill or disabled through support groups, caregiver networks, and a bimonthly newsletter.

Other Helpful Resources
Books
Beyond Chaos: One Man's Journey Alongside His Chronically Ill Wife by Gregg Piburn

Caregiver's Reprieve: A Guide to Emotional Survival When You're Caring for Someone You Love by Avrene L. Brandt

The Caregiving Wife's Handbook by Diana Denholm

Chronic Illness and the Family: A Guide to Living Every Day by Dr. Linda Welsh and Marian Betancourt

Kind Words for Caring People: Daily Affirmations for Caregivers by Sefra Kobrin Pitzele

Online Magazines and Websites with Chat Groups
Caregiver-Information.com
www.caregiver-information.com

Caregiver Partnership
www.caregiverpartnership.com/resources/categories

Caregiving.com
www.caregiving.com

Caregiving Resources
www.caregivingresources.com

Careguide.com
www.careguide.com

Healthy Caregiver.com
www.healthycaregiver.com

Today's Caregiver Magazine Online
www.caregiver.com

Counseling and Psychology Resources

American Psychological Association Referral Service
http://locator.apa.org

British Psychological Society
www.bps.org.uk

CRPS/RSD Organizations and Online Groups

American RSDHope
www.rsdhope.org

Australian RSD Group
www.ozrsd.org/web/main.htm

Ayala's No Pain Zone
www.nopainzone.com

Belgian Support Group for Patients with Sudeck's Atrophy
www.zelfhulp.be/zoek/index.php?boxaction=toonprobleem&prob
leem=ALGONEURODYSTROFIE

Belgian information on RSD/support-group contacts
http://users.skynet.be/d.lineate/crps/zelfhulp_EN.html

Fighting 4 Us
http://fighting4us.com

German RSD Support Group
www.shz-muenchen.de/index.php?m=2&id=293

Healthboards Patient Support Forum (RSD)
www.healthboards.com/boards/reflex-sympathetic-dystrophy-rsd
-crps

International Research Foundation for RSD/CRPS
www.rsdinfo.com/AboutRSD.htm

Nederlandse Vereniging van Post-Traumatische Patienten
www.posttraumatischedystrofie.nl/

Neurotalk Online Patient Support Room (RSD and CRPS)
http://neurotalk.psychcentral.com/forum21.html

Promoting Awareness of RSD and CRPS in Canada (PARC)
www.rsdcanada.org/parc/english

Reflex Sympathetic Dystrophy Syndrome Association of America (RSDSA)
www.rsds.org

RSD Aware
www.rsdawareness.com

RSD-CRPS United Kingdom
www.rsd-crps.co.uk

RSD/CRPS World News Group
http://health.groups.yahoo.com/group/RSD-WorldNews

RSD Hope for Kids Under 14
www.angelfire.com/my/rsdhopekids/index.html

RSD Hope for Teens 14 and Up
www.angelfire.com/wi/rsdhopeteens

RSD Parent Group
http://groups.yahoo.com/group/RSDParents

South Carolina RSD Association
www.scrsda.org

Disability Support Resources

American Association of People with Disabilities
2013 H St. NW, 5th Fl.
Washington DC 20006
(800) 840-8844
(202) 457-0046 voice/TTY
www.aapd.com

Canadian Abilities Foundation
http://abilities.ca

Contact a Family
209-211 City Rd.
London
EC1V 1JN
020 7608 8700
Helpline: 0808 808 3555
www.cafamily.org.uk
A British charity providing support and advice to parents with an ill child.

Job Resources for People with Disabilities
American Association of People with Disabilities (AAPD)
http://jobs.aapd.com/jobs

Disability Employment Resources
www.gladnet.org

Disability Resources Monthly
www.disabilityresources.org

Hire Potential
www.hirepotential.com

Job Accommodation Network
http://janweb.icdi.wvu.edu
A free consulting service that provides information about job accommodations, the Americans with Disabilities Act (ADA), and the employability of people with disabilities.

Office of Personnel Management: Federal Jobs for Disabled Workers
www.opm.gov/policy-data-oversight/disability-employment/getting-a -job

National Business and Disability Council
www.business-disability.com/Job_Seekers/job_seekers.asp

The Work Site
www.socialsecurity.gov/work

General Pain Organizations and Resources

American Academy of Pain Management
www.aapainmanage.org

American Academy of Pain Medicine
www.painmed.org

American Chronic Pain Association
www.theacpa.org

American Pain Society
www.ampainsoc.org

American Society of Interventional Pain Physicians
www.asipp.org

Australian Pain Society
www.apsoc.org.au

British Pain Society
www.britishpainsociety.org

Canadian Chronic Pain Society
http://chronicpaincanada.com

Canadian Pain Society
www.canadianpainsociety.ca

European Pain
www.efic.org (European division of IASP)

For Grace
www.forgrace.org

International Association for the Study of Pain (IASP)
www.pain.com
The IASP has a subcommittee, Special Interest Group on Pain and the Sympathetic Nervous System.

National Organization of Rare Disorders
www.rarediseases.org

New Zealand Pain Society
www.nzps.org.nz

Medical and Pharmaceutical Resources

Compounding Pharmacies

FDA Information on Compounding Pharmacies
www.fda.gov/Drugs/GuidanceComplianceRegulatoryInformation/PharmacyCompounding/default.htm (Overview)
www.fda.gov/Drugs/GuidanceComplianceRegulatoryInformation/PharmacyCompounding/ucm339771.htm (Warnings on Recalls)

International Academy of Compounding Pharmacists
www.iacprx.org

Find Medical Professionals and Pain Clinics

http://crpsadvisory.com/crpsa_pain_management_and_frp.html#.Uq TjwfRDskw
www.doctordirectory.com
www.findadoc.com
www.healthgrades.com
www.medicinenet.com/pain_management/city.htm

pain.com/pain-clinic

www.partnersagainstpain.com/pain-management-resources/tips.aspx

Hospital Protocol for Handling CRPS/RSD Patients
www.rsds.org/4/resources/pdf/hospital_protocol.pdf

MedicAlert Foundation
(800) 633-4298

www.medicalert.org

MedicAlert can store your unique medical information and provide you with a medical bracelet to wear, so doctors check them first for guidance in case of emergency.

Prescription Assistance Programs
www.medicare.gov/pharmaceutical-assistance-program/index.aspx

www.pparx.org

www.rxassist.org

Recognizing Medical "Quacks" or Fraud
United States: www.quackwatch.com

Canada: www.healthwatcher.net/Quackerywatch/index.html

Mobility and Transportation

Adaptive Mobility Services

www.adaptivemobility.com

Community Transportation Association of America

www.ctaa.org

Hope Air of Canada

www.hopeair.org

Arranges free air transportation for Canadians who must travel to obtain medical care, but cannot afford the flight costs. They will arrange international flights if the medical care cannot be obtained in Canada.

National Patient Travel Center

www.PatientTravel.org

Provides a variety of services to those seeking a way to travel long distances for specialized medical evaluation, diagnosis, and treatment. The National Patient Travel HELPLINE can be reached at (800) 296-1217.

Recommended Reading

General

Bauby, Jean-Dominique. *The Diving Bell and the Butterfly* (New York: Vintage Press, 1998).

Benson, Ann, and Rebecca Carter. *The Encyclopedia of Craft Projects for the First Time* (New York: Sterling Publishing, 2002).

Benson, Herbert with William Proctor. *Beyond the Relaxation Response* (New York: Berkley Publishing Group, 1985).

Berg, Art. *The Impossible Just Takes a Little Longer* (New York: Quill, 2003).

Brandt, Avrene L. *Caregiver's Reprieve: A Guide to Emotional Survival when You're Caring for Someone You Love* (Atascadero, CA: Impact Publishers, 1997).

Buff, Sheila. *Birding for Beginners* (Guilford, CT: The Lyons Press, 1993).

Carrico, Mara, and the editors of *Yoga Journal*. *Yoga Journal's Yoga Basics: the Essential Guide to Yoga for a Lifetime of Health and Fitness* (New York: Owl Books, 1997).

Caudill, Margaret. *Managing Pain Before It Manages You* (New York: Guilford Press, 1994).

Christensen, Alice. *The American Yoga Association's Easy Does It Yoga: The Safe and Gentle Way to Health and Well-Being* (New York: Fireside Books, 1999).

Das, Lama Surya. *Letting Go of the Person You Used to Be* (New York: Broadway Books, 2003).

Davies, Clair. *The Trigger Point Therapy Workbook: Your Self-Treatment Guide for Pain Relief* (Oakland, CA: New Harbinger, 2001).

Hanh, Thich Nhat. *Being Peace* (Berkeley, CA: Parallax Press, 1987).

Hinds, Erv. *A Life Larger than Pain* (Albuquerque, NM: Health Press, 2003).

Kabat-Zinn, Jon. *Full Catastrophe Living: Using the Wisdom of Your Body and Mind to Face Stress, Pain, and Illness* (New York: Delta Trade Paperbacks, 1990).

Kabat-Zinn, Jon. *Mindfulness Meditation for Pain Relief: Guided Practices for Reclaiming Your Body and Your Life.*

Iyengar, B. K. S. *Yoga: The Path to Holistic Health* (New York: DK Publishing, 2001).

Lee Johnson, Yanling. *Qigong for Living* (Roslindale, MA: YMAA Publication Center, 2002).

Lindsay, Terence, and R. G. Turner. *Backyard Birding* (Chain Sales Marketing, Inc., 2002).

National Geographic Field Guide to the Birds of North America, 4th edition (Roanoke, VA: National Geographic Society, 2002).

Piburn, Gregg. *Beyond Chaos: One Man's Journey Alongside His Chronically Ill Wife* (The Arthritis Foundation, 1999).

Pitzele, Sefra Kobrin. *Kind Words for Caring People: Daily Affirmations for Caregivers* (Deerfield Beach, FL: Health Communications, 1992).

Simons, David, Janet Travell, Lois Simons, and Barbara Cummings. *Travell and Simons' Myofascial Pain and Dysfunction: The Trigger Point Manual.* (Philadelphia, PA: Lippincott, Williams & Wilkins, 1998).

Storr, Anthony. *Solitude: A Return to the Self* (New York: Ballantine Books, 1989).

Welsh, Linda, and Marian Betancourt. *Chronic Illness and the Family: A Guide to Living Every Day* (Avon, MA: Adams Media Corporation, 1996).

Werner, Doug. *Backpacker's Start-Up: A Beginner's Guide to Hiking & Backpacking* (Chula Vista, CA: Tracks Publishing, 1999).

Books Written by CRPS Patients

Ingle, Barby. *RSD in Me! A Patient and Caretaker Guide to Reflex Sympathetic Dystrophy and Other Chronic Pain Conditions* (Self-published, 2009).

Lang, Linda. *Living with RSDS: Your Guide to Coping with Reflex Sympathetic Dystrophy Syndrome* (Oakland, CA: New Harbinger Publications, 2003).

Toussaint, Cynthia. *Battle for Grace: A Memoir of Pain, Redemption and Impossible Love* (Self-published, 2003).

Solutions for Limited or No Health Insurance
www.coverageforall.org/resources
www.healthcare.gov
www.insurekidsnow.gov/state

Wellness Organizations and Resources
Many of these websites include directories to allow users to search for a practitioner in their region.

Acupuncture
American Association of Acupuncture & Oriental Medicine
www.aaaomonline.org

World Federation of Acupuncture—Moxibustion Societies
www.wfas.org.cn/en

Art Therapy
American Art Therapy Association
www.arttherapy.org

Biofeedback
Association for Applied Psychophysiology and Biofeedback
www.aapb.org

Biofeedback Certification Institute of America
www.bcia.org

Calmare (Scrambler Therapy)
www.calmarett.com

Complementary Medicine
National Center for Complementary and Alternative Medicine
www.nccam.nih.gov

Craniosacral Therapy
Find a Craniosacral Therapist
www.iahp.com/pages/search/index.php

Craniosacral Association of the United Kingdom
www.craniosacral.co.uk

Feldenkrais
Feldenkrais Guild of North America
www.feldenkrais.com

Find a Feldenkrais Practitioner Worldwide
www.feldenkraisguild.com/find

Homeopathy
British Institute of Homeopathy
www.britinsthom.com

European Council of Classic Homeopathy
www.homeopathy-ecch.org

North American Society for Homeopaths
http://homeopathy.org

Hyperbaric Oxygen Therapy
Undersea and Hyperbaric Medical Society
www.uhms.org

Hypnosis/Hypnotherapy
American Association of Professional Hypnotherapists
http://aaph.org

Canadian Hypnotherapy Association
http://www.canadianhypnotherapyassociation.ca

Light Therapy
Low-Level Laser Therapy Association Links
www.laser.nu/lllt/llltorganisation.htm

Massage Therapy
American Massage Therapy Association
www.amtamassage.org

Australian Association of Massage Therapists
www.amt.org.au

Canadian Massage Therapy Alliance
www.cmta.ca

Meditation Resources
Mindfulness Meditation for Pain Relief: Guided Practices for Reclaiming Your Body and Your Life by Jon Kabat-Zinn

Guided Mindfulness Unabridged on 4 CDs, by Jon Kabat-Zinn
www.guidedimageryinc.com

Free Guided Meditations, UCLA Mindful Awareness Resource Center
http://marc.ucla.edu/body.cfm?id=22

University of Massachusetts Medical School Center for Mindfulness
www.umassmed.edu/Content.aspx?id=41254&amp

The World Wide Online Meditation Center
www.meditationcenter.com

Naturopathy
American Naturopathic Medical Association
www.anma.org

Canadian Associations of Naturopathic Doctors
www.naturopathicassoc.ca

Neurological Disorders
National Institute of Neurological Disorders and Stroke
www.ninds.nih.gov

Occupational Therapy
American Occupational Therapy Association
www.aota.org

Canadian Association of Occupational Therapists
www.caot.ca

Osteopathy
American Osteopathic Association
www.aoa-net.org

Physical Therapy
American Physical Therapy Association
www.apta.org

Canadian Physiotherapy Association
www.physiotherapy.ca

Qigong
American Qigong Association
www.nqa.org

Reiki
International Reiki Alliance
www.reikialliance.com/en

Thermal Imaging/Thermography
American Academy of Medical Infrared Imaging
http://aathermology.org

Yoga
Books
American Yoga Association's Easy Does It Yoga: The Safe and Gentle Way to Health and Well-Being by Alice Christensen

Yoga Journal's Yoga Basics: The Essential Guide to Yoga for a Lifetime of Health and Fitness by Mara Carrico and the editors of Yoga Journal

Yoga: The Path to Holistic Health by B. K. S. Iyengar

Organizations
Kripalu Yoga Teachers Association and Library
http://kripalu.org

Videos
Bedtop Yoga by Carol Dickman

Gentle Kripalu by William Swotes

Seated Yoga by Carol Dickman

Zero-Balancing
Zero-Balancing Health Association
www.zerobalancing.com

Index